PRAISE FOR C⟨⟩ W9-AGG-250

The Healing Powers of Olive Oil, Revised and Updated

"One of the most healing foods on the planet. A fascinating read—olive oil is not only delicious—it is good medicine!"
—Ann Louise Gittleman, Ph.D.

"Orey gives kudos to olive oil—and people of all ages will benefit from her words of wisdom."
—Dr. Will Clower, CEO, Mediterranean Wellness

"Olive oil has been known for centuries to have healing powers and now we know why. It is rich in monounsaturated fats similar to avocado and macadamia nut oils. The information in this book will help you to understand the healing powers of oils."
—Fred Pescatore, M.D., M.P.H., author of *The Hamptons Diet*

The Healing Powers of Olive Oil

"Olive oil is one of our important foods. This book deserves to be in everybody's home library."
—Elson M. Haas, M.D., author of *Staying Healthy with Nutrition, 21st Century Edition*

"A fascinating read about olive oil's secret ingredients."
—Chef Ann Cooper, author of *Lunch Lessons: Changing the Way We Feed Our Children*

"This is a landmark book, full of entertaining anecdotes, which explains the olive oil and health connections."
—Jan McBarron, M.D.

The Healing Powers of Coffee

"A cup or two of joe every day is a good way to boost mood, energy, and overall health."
>—Julian Whitaker, M.D., founder of the
>Whitaker Wellness Institute

"For heart, mind, and body, Cal Orey shows us why coffee is the most comforting health food on the planet."
>—Dr. Will Clower, CEO Mediterranean Wellness

"All of the Healing Powers books have been widely popular on our network of thousands of food bloggers. Her latest book on coffee is no exception!"
>—Jenn Campus, cofounder of the Foodie Blogroll

The Healing Powers of Honey

"Cal Orey scores again with *The Healing Powers of Honey*, a continuation of her widely praised Healing Powers series. Orey's honey book is well researched in a manner that makes it both entertaining and informative. This book will make you look at honey in a new way—as a bona fide health food as well as a gastronomic treat."
>—Joe Traynor, author of *Honey: The Gourmet Medicine*

"Not everyone can be a beekeeper, but Cal Orey shares the secrets that honeybees and their keepers have always known. Honey is good for body and soul."
>—Kim Flottum, editor of *Bee Culture* magazine and
>author of several honeybee books

The Healing Powers of Chocolate

"This book blends my favorite two things: chocolate and romance (not necessarily in that order). This book will rev up your romance and titillate your sensibilities. Treat yourself and your partner to all the truth about chocolate that's fit to print!"
—Larry James, wedding officiant, author

"Chocolate is a taste of divine ecstasy on Earth. It is our sensual communion. Orey's journalistic style and efforts share this insight with readers around the world."
—Jim Walsh, founder of Intentional Chocolate

The Healing Powers of Vinegar

"A practical, health-oriented book that everyone who wants to stay healthy and live longer should read."
—Patricia Bragg, N.D., Ph.D., author of *Apple Cider Vinegar*

"Deserves to be included in everybody's kitchen and medicine chest."
—Ann Louise Gittleman, Ph.D.

"Wonderfully useful for everyone interested in health."
—Elson M. Haas, M.D., author of *Staying Healthy with Nutrition,* 21st *Century Edition*

Books by Cal Orey

The Healing Powers of Vinegar
Doctors' Orders
202 Pets' Peeves
The Healing Powers of Olive Oil
The Healing Powers of Chocolate
The Healing Powers of Honey
The Healing Powers of Coffee

Published by Kensington Publishing Corporation

THE HEALING POWERS OF

Olive Oil

A Complete Guide to Nature's Liquid Gold

REVISED AND UPDATED

CAL OREY

KENSINGTON BOOKS
www.kensingtonbooks.com

Permission to reproduce The Mediterranean Pyramid Diet Pyramid and Common Foods and Flavors of the Mediterranean Diet Pyramid © 2009, granted by Oldways Preservation & Exchange Trust, www.oldwayspt.org.

KENSINGTON BOOKS are published by

Kensington Publishing Corp.
119 West 40th Street
New York, NY 10018

Copyright © 2008, 2015 by Cal Orey

All rights reserved. No part of this book may be reproduced in any form or by any means without the prior written consent of the Publisher, excepting brief quotes used in reviews.

If you purchased this book without a cover, you should be aware that this book is stolen property. It was reported as "unsold and destroyed" to the Publisher amd neither the Author nor the Publisher has received any payment for this "stripped book."

All Kensington Titles, Imprints and Distributed Lines are available at special quantity discounts for bulk purchases for sales promotions, premiums, fund-raising, and educational or institutional use. Special book excerpts or customized printings can also be created to fit specific needs. For details, write or phone the office of the Kensington special sales manager: Kensington Publishing Corp., 119 West 40th Street, New York, NY 10018, attn: Special Sales Department, Phone: 1-800-221-2647.

Kensington and the K logo Reg. U.S. Pat & TM Off.

ISBN-13: 978-1-4967-0384-2
ISBN-10: 1-4967-0384-7
First Kensington Trade Paperback Edition: February 2008
First Kensington Mass Market Edition: January 2009
Revised and Updated Trade Edition: January 2015
Revised and Updated Mass Market Edition: January 2016

eISBN-13: 978-1-4967-0385-9
eISBN-10: 1-4967-0385-5
Kensington Electronic Edition: January 2016
10 9 8 7 6 5 4 3 2 1

Printed in the United States of America

This book is intended as a reference tool only. It does not give medical advice. Be sure to consult your health care practitioner before starting any diet or exercise program.

I dedicate this book to the olive tree. I am connected to the hardy, productive olive tree groves in my native state of California; in Italy, Spain, Greece; and around the globe. The universal superfood and its healing versatile virtues are a blessing to the well-being of people of all ages.

CONTENTS

Foreword

IN THE LAND OF OLIVE OIL

The same thing happened to me twice, in two different cities. The first time was at a book signing in Cleveland, Ohio, when a small woman came straight up to me and asked, "Can you guess how old I am?"

She looked like she was about 68 to 72ish (and I know how this game works), so I guessed low. "Oh gosh, no more than 65," I responded.

She straightened up just a little bit taller and said, "I'm 88 years old."

This woman was stunning. Her skin was perfect, and she just radiated health. I said, "Okay, WHAT? What are you doing?"

She told me that she was a first-generation Italian, her family consumed olive oil every day, and her mother even put it right on her skin. Every day!

The Healthiest Diet on Earth

We look at cases like this, as does author Cal Orey, and wonder how in the world they knew to do that. But the knowledge that the rich, delicious oil of the olive will keep them younger and more vibrant for more of their days doesn't come from some laboratory. They don't do it because some science study told them to.

The knowledge they rely upon, like the rich, multilayered

complexity of olive oil itself, comes from the ancient cultural traditions of these thin, healthy people. There is a depth to that cultural understanding, which also forms the centerpiece to what many deem the healthiest diet on earth: the olive oil–based Mediterranean diet.

Could you imagine someone from Spain or Greece exclaiming how they suddenly weren't going to eat olive oil because some study came out about low-fat foods? That would be ridiculous. Or perhaps they'd turn to a low-fat dressing because they read that the ratio of hydrogens saturating its fatty acid chain didn't fit some theory about what should or shouldn't constitute a healthy oil. Absurd.

The thin, healthy people consumed olive oil when scientists recommended against it and continue this delicious habit after scientists embraced it. Their dietary prescriptions haven't changed precisely because the decision to eat olive oil is an expression of who they are as a people.

There is a steady depth to this form of cultural knowledge, embedded in the steady passage of time across ages. It's an expression of who they are, who their parents are, extending across time like an outstretched hand to us today, directly from their history, culture, and tradition.

Because of this solid foundation, you can count on it to work for your good health, just as well as it has worked for theirs.

After all, it has done so since before history was written down and won't change in the next five years either. The impact on your health will be the same as it has been felt for millennia. And when you look at the results over this expanse of time, you see that olive oil consumption is clearly associated with low weight, healthy hearts, and longer lives.

The people of Crete, for example, as I know and Orey pointed out in the first edition of *The Healing Powers of Olive Oil*, have some of the highest longevity rates on Earth, some of the lowest cardiac mortality rates and cancer rates, and all with the highest per capita consumption of olive oil. Ask them about their amazing heart-healthy diet and they'll shrug because they're not on a diet. They're just living their lives as they always have.

It's strange, too, that the remarkable health benefits of olive oil have been known to people in the Mediterranean region for millennia, but the rest of the world is just now catching up with them. With each month, it seems, new scientific research continually reconfirms the many ways in which it benefits our bodies.

OLIVE OIL, THE VERSATILE FAT

Orey, once again, in *The Healing Powers of Olive Oil, Revised and Updated*, with the greatest of ease, explains the fats in olive oil that we feared for so long turn out to be the monounsaturated and polyunsaturated variety, which today's science confirms can help reduce your risk of heart disease.

The antioxidants found within the deep green oil also work inside your body to fight the harmful free radicals. On your salad, in your sauté, or simply drizzled over your fish, this helps prevent cellular damage and, ultimately, the development of cancer itself.

Not only are these amazing fats good for you on their own, but they can also help your body absorb the other healthful nutrients in your food, such as the fat soluble vitamins A, D, E, and K. In other words, if you include olive oil on any of your foods, you get one health enhancement from the olive oil, and then a turbo boost from the added nutrients you absorb from your salad.

The cultural habit of applying olive oil both inside and out, for softer, smoother, less desiccated skin, has been known and practiced for thousands of years. Now our Western science confirms that the dermal application of olive oil leaves your skin less dry, less wrinkled, and less susceptible to DNA damage caused by exposure to UV light.

THE SUPERFOOD THAT'S GOOD AS GOLD

So whether you are a person who needs science to quantify and verify what you see in order to believe it, or someone who trusts what healthy cultures are doing and can apply those habits to your own life, the jury is pretty much in on olive oil. It's great for you!

Cal Orey's *The Healing Powers of Olive Oil: A Complete Guide to Nature's Liquid Gold, Revised and Updated* clearly lays out more research and more reasons why olive oil (also paired with other healing oils) is healthy, how you can use it, which kind is the best, where you can find it, and many delicious ways you can incorporate it into your daily life, for added flavor, better health, and even beauty! Orey gives credit to olive oil—and people will benefit from her words of wisdom.

—Dr. Will Clower, CEO, Mediterranean Wellness, and award-winning author of *The Fat Fallacy* and *Eat Chocolate, Lose Weight*

Acknowledgments

I admit that when I wrote the first edition of *The Healing Powers of Olive Oil*, I was clueless about olive oil and its amazing health merits and other precious cooking oils—all types—so it was a foreign topic for me. Special thanks to passionate olive oil masters, including the North American Olive Oil Association, Nick Sciabica & Sons, The Olive Press, medical doctors, and researchers who inspired me, a health author, and my taste buds to revisit Olive Oil Land.

The tide is changing in the twenty-first century when it comes to using healing oils. I confess I wasn't always an olive oil lover. During research of the original book, I didn't know porcini oil from citrus olive oil, or that Spain was and still is the largest olive oil producer in the world. But I was an eager student. And, in the new edition, gratitude goes, too, to the companies who shared their products and worldly knowledge of both olive oil (all types) and other healing oils making headway in the health world.

This second time around, I went on a new expedition into the wide world of olive oils (cooking and baking with them) and learned how to use different cooking oils, too, for heart health, longevity, home cures, and beauty aids. I braved the uncharted land and tried myriad cooking oils—not just extra virgin olive oil.

Also, I recall receiving e-mails from a bold fan—challenging me about fat facts. She agreed that while olive oil is healthy, I should give more credit to saturated fat (including butter and cheese). New research has shown me that the "un"-fats like monounsaturated and polyunsaturated fats aren't the only ones that are good for us. I give thanks to my dear reader who was spot-on and gave me incentive to dig deeper to find the truth in the ever changing world of food and health. So to prepare this second edition, I went back to the drawing board. I discovered during my journey that indulging in other oils like coconut oil and macadamia oil (which do contain saturated fat) and even decadent butter boasts health perks. And it's time to give appreciation to these ignored newbies and comeback oldies, too.

Also, since I'm fessing up, the fact is I was "sneaking" foods like butter in my diet, but I didn't tell my devout olive oil contacts and friends. But my instincts told me that by pairing a bit of the forbidden fat with olive oils it made my cookies, cakes, and entrées taste better and felt good inside and outside my body. And that's when I pushed my olive oils over on my pantry shelves and made room for other healing oils (including nut and tropical)—and I'm glad I did it.

These days, as a devout Food Network junkie (America's television food channel) and accidental health-nut foodie, I thank chefs, including Emeril Lagasse, who use both olive oil and other cooking oils and butter (all kinds). For years now, I've been using both the oil and fat together, and now I no longer feel guilty about combining olive oil and butter to enjoy my dishes more.

Finally, I have been blessed with an enthusiastic editor who asked me to go back and revise and update my second Healing Powers series book on olive oil. In an olive seed, once again, I got to explore the olive oil and cooking oils world from the comfort of my cabin in the California Sierra—through changing seasons. The best part is, as a baby boomer (a person born between 1946 and 1964), I now have a new, improved relationship with healing oils. I sense this book, like the first one, was meant to get a makeover by me for you. A toast to olive oil—and other healing oils—is as good as it gets.

Author's Note

A word on measuring: At King Arthur Flour, the bakers believe measuring ingredients by weight (ounces) is more accurate than measuring by volume (cups and spoons). But since the volume system is still standard, they use it along with weight measurements. You may use either in their recipes included in this book.

Real recipes, tried and true: The recipes in this book have been tested by me, and/or veteran chefs, bakers, and olive oil experts. But note that changing ingredients or using different kitchen tools or methods may alter taste, texture, and presentation of a dish. Plus, culinary palates vary.

PART 1

A Time for Olive Oil

1

The Power of Olive Oil

Except the vine, there is no plant which bears a fruit of as great importance as the olive.

—Pliny[1]

I was born and raised in Umbria, Italy, on my family's ancient olive plantation. My father was half Irish, a fair-skinned, redheaded, stocky, sturdy, hardworking olive grove farmer. My mother, a petite, dark-haired Italian woman with piercing blue eyes, ran a charming bed-and-breakfast cottage. She served and sold homemade bread, cheese, vegetables, fruit, and olive oil. The days were long, but our fruits of labor were worth the efforts for the well-being of our family, the community, and the tourists who liked our cozy, rustic lifestyle on the Mediterranean.

One overcast, cool November morning in the kitchen with my mom, I learned the art of baking drop scones. I forgot to include the pale yellow liquid gold. My detail-oriented mother, a seasoned baker, mumbled, "Tsk-tsk" as she poured the liquid gold into the thick batter. When the scones were baked and the fruity scent filled the air of the kitchen, she dipped a warm scone full of olives and nuts into a beautifully decorated olive oil dish. She smiled and handed me the treat as a truce. In the real world, this rural picturesque scene is a dream of mine. While I would love to be an olive farmer's daughter living in Europe, the truth of the matter is it's not the real story of my roots.

In the fifties, I grew up in San Jose, California, a place once known for its plentiful prune tree orchards. Today, as a nature-loving Northern Californian who currently lives amid tall pine trees in South Lake Tahoe, I was pleasantly surprised to discover that within three hours of my mountain-style home—with rolling hills much like in Italy, Spain, and Greece—olive groves are growing and people are producing olive oil, known as liquid gold (coined centuries ago) in Mediterranean-type weather in the Golden State.

When I was in my late twenties, it was my dream to go to Europe. I dog-eared one of those Europe-on-a-shoestring-budget travel books and planned my trip. But I opted to go to graduate school instead. So, I never got to enjoy the exotic Mediterranean countries or taste the European cuisine—including its wide world of olive oil.

The closest I've come to Italy, the second largest producer of olive oil, is by watching the film *Under the Tuscan Sun*, which is about a divorced writing professor and book reviewer—played by Diane Lane—and based loosely on a novel created by Frances Mayes, who taught classes at my alumni college, San Francisco State University. With envy, I viewed her protagonist, Frances, learning to live and laugh again thousands of miles away from the San Francisco Bay Area. In Tuscany, where she relocates, it's the eccentric, down-to-earth locals and observing an earthy harvest of olives (right outside her new home) that finds a place in her heart.

In the real world, I sit here in my study with a melting winter snow-covered ground outdoors in the California Sierras and fantasize about how wonderful it would be to live in Italy amid olive trees. But, whisking off in a plane to Europe isn't going to happen for me today or tomorrow. Still, I will take you along with me to visit real people and real places where you will get a real flavor of the Mediterranean basin and of the healing powers of olive oil.

THE OLIVE YIELDS A POWERFUL OIL

Olive oil has been praised by people as one of Mother Nature's most healthful fats, especially if it is extra virgin olive oil. And now, olive oil—and other healing oils—are making the news worldwide, and are here to stay in homes, restaurants, and even fast-food chains.

People from all walks of life—including some olive oil pioneers and contemporary medical experts—believe olive oil helps fight body fat and keeps blood pressure down as well as heart disease at bay. Olive oil is also known to help relieve colds and maintain healthy skin.

These days, well-known health gurus continue to tout olive oil, a timeless superfood, as have others I have mentioned in the past. I watched Dr. Mehmet Oz, for one, on *The Dr. Oz Show* praise liquid gold—and avocado oil to coconut oil. Chefs—not just Rachael Ray—use olive oil paired with other oils and fats in an array of dishes. And other masters of food and health have applauded the timeless benefits of olive oil, too.

Jean Carper, a leading authority on health and nutrition, points out that new Italian research finds olive oil contains antioxidants, similar to those in tea and red wine, that fight heart disease, including LDL cholesterol's ability to clog arteries.[2]

Dietician and nutrition consultant Pat Baird, author of *The Pyramid Cookbook: Pleasures of the Food Guide Pyramid*, touts the golden liquid, too. "I love the whole idea of olive oil's versatility. I use it for baking, as well as salad dressings and sautéing. Olive oil has been around for a long time, and the more we know about it, the more we learn about its great contribution to good health."[3]

Liz Applegate, Ph.D., a renowned health, nutrition, and fitness expert, wrote in her book *101 Miracle Foods That Heal Your Heart*, "Rich in history, and even richer in heart-healthy benefits, olive oil is the 'king' of oils."[4]

Health-Boosting Nutrients in Extra Virgin Olive Oil

Medical researchers around the world continue to find new health-promoting nutrients in olives and olive oil. Here are some of the nutrients in extra virgin olive oil:

Vitamin E: an antioxidant vitamin that can help strengthen immune responses and reduce the risk of heart disease and some forms of cancer.

Essential Fatty Acids: good-for-you fats such as the healthy balance of omega-3s and omega-6s that can help stave off heart disease, obesity, and diabetes.

Chlorophyll: a substance that has antioxidant properties.

Phenol Compounds: substances that also act as antioxidants.

Phytoestrogens: substances that may help beat bone loss and minimize pesky symptoms of menopause.

Sterols: substances that counter the intestinal absorption of cholesterol in foods.

Most important, like apple cider and red wine vinegars, extra virgin olive oil contains polyphenols, naturally occurring compounds that act as powerful antioxidants (disease-fighting enzymes that protect your body by trapping free-radical molecules and getting rid of them before damage occurs).

OLIVE OILS WITH POLYPHENOLS

Keep in mind, if you're a health-conscious person like I try to be, you'll quickly ask, "Which olive oil has the highest polyphenols?"

"Phenol content is determined by olive variety, time of picking, olive condition and processing method, whether the oil is refined, and the length of time the oil has been treated," explains Dr. John Deane, an internal medicine specialist in Marin County, California, and an olive oil expert who founded and used to write articles for *The Olive Oil Source* newsletter.

That said, it's the Tuscan varieties, points out Deane, such as Coratina, Frantoio, Lucca, and Pendolino, that boast the highest good-for-you polyphenols. "These oils are valuable in that when blended with a low polyphenol oil, they will extend the shelf life by preventing rancidity," he adds.

The olive oil master also says that the bulk of olive oil we consume in America comes from Italy and Spain. But the glitch is, that means it's most likely refined—and lower in phenols.

So, what do you do if you're on a mission to get an olive oil that is polyphenol-rich? According to Deane, if you choose a brand that reads "extra virgin," boasts the California Olive Oil Council (COOC) seal, is from the "current harvest season," and has been properly stored, you should be holding a healthful bottle of olive oil, like a good bottle of antioxidant-rich wine, with polyphenols.

Another interesting note I discovered is that olive oils that are higher in polyphenols tend to be harsher, bitter, and stronger flavored. That makes me think of dark chocolate. It is not as sweet and mellow as milk chocolate. But then, it's the darker chocolate that contains the heart-healthy antioxidants, right? And, like other healthful foods, such as olive oil, sometimes it takes a while to acquire a taste for them.

OLIVE OIL BASICS 101

Olive oil, one of the oldest vegetable oils, comes from the fruit of the olive tree *(Olea europae L.)*, which was originally found in the Mediterranean basin. It has been used since biblical times in cooking, as a medicinal agent, in cosmetics, in soaps, and even as fuel for lamps.

So, what exactly is olive oil, anyhow?

Olive Oil: oil pressed from olives, used in salad dressings, for cooking, as an ingredient in soaps, and as an emollient.
—*The American Heritage Dictionary*

Olive oil can be made from a wide variety of olives, such as black and green olives, and other types. "There are at least

30 olive varieties used extensively for olive oil and then add another 100 or so depending on where you are. In total, 300-plus varieties," explains Judy Ridgway, an olive oil guru based in the United Kingdom. Of course, I have learned that this number varies depending on your olive oil reference source.

The following kinds of olives—including the polyphenol-rich ones—used for olive oils are listed from A to Z, with guidance from olive oil wizard Ridgway.

OLIVE POTPOURRI

Kind	Olives Grown From	Olive Oil Taste
Arbequina	Puglia, Italy	Fresh and fruity
Barnea	Australia, Israel, New Zealand	Sweet almonds, sometimes with a banana flavor
Biancollia	Sicily	Herbal tomatoes
Cerasuolo	Sicily	Apples, sweet herbs, and tomatoes
Coratina	Carato (near Barl) and Puglia, Italy	Fruity, bitter, and peppery with a tinge of sweet taste; high in polyphenols
Cornicabra	Spain	Light bitterness, peppery, and fruit notes; younger oils pungent, smooth, like an almond aftertaste

Kind	Olives Grown From	Olive Oil Taste
Frantoio	Tuscany, Italy; Argentina; Chile; California; New Zealand; Australia	Fruity, aromatic, and a peppery taste; late bloomers soft, almost sweet, like a mild almond flavor
Galega	Portugal	Fruity smell, soft, smooth flavor of green fruit and grass with a taste of almonds
Hojblanca	Andalusia, Spain	Often sweet, and a bit fruity, followed by a mild peppery taste; a lingering bitter aftertaste of fruit
Kalamata	Kalamata, Greece	Distinct taste
Koroneiki	Koroni, Greece	Fruity, touch of green apple, fresh, grassy flavor
La Tanche	Nyons, Provence, France; Sicily	Sweet apples and herbs
Leccino	Tuscany, Umbria, Lazio, Italy	Bland, a bit fruity, not bitter or peppery, a little sweetness
Maurino	Central Italy and California	Bitter herbs with nuts and pepper

Kind	Olives Grown From	Olive Oil Taste
Mission	California	Fruity, more peppery and bitter than Cornicabra oils, thick, a hint of almond sweetness
Moraiolo	Central Italy	Herbaceous with bitter nuts and pepper
Nocellara Del Belice	Castelvetrano, Italy	Fresh and delightful flavor
Ogilarolo	Puglia, Italy	Sweet nuts and light apples
Olivastra	Tuscany and Slovenia	Creamy apples and herbs
Peranzana	Southern Italy	Herbs and bitter salad leaves
Picholine	France	Lacks bitterness, mild, almost sweet
Picual	Spain	Distinct [butter] and strong taste like "figs and wet wood"; high polyphenols
Picudo	Spain	Smooth, strong, and distinctive taste; sweet; grassy first; strong aroma of bitter citrus; low levels of polyphenols

Kind	Olives Grown From	Olive Oil Taste
Taggiasca	Liguria, Italy	Sweet apples, nuts, and light herbs
Tonda Iblea	Sicily	Crushed tomatoes

THE ART OF PRODUCTION

From harvesting to bottling, the time and tender loving care put into nature's olives and making premium quality olive oil is the same today as it was centuries ago. In the twenty-first century, olive oil is made in Mediterranean countries such as Spain, Italy, and Greece, and a percentage is produced in California, Australia, parts of South America, and other countries from Brazil to China.

Harvesting: Varying from region to region, olive harvests usually take place between mid-November and mid-January. During this time, olive oil producers are much like writers on deadline—busy, excited, and did I say busy? The olives are collected in nets that are placed around the foot of the tree (see the film *Under the Tuscan Sun* to get a visual image), and within 24 hours of harvest, the olives are taken directly to a mill to be pressed into olive oil.

Pressing: An olive paste is created by crushing the whole fruit (yes, including the pits that you spit out when munching on your favorite olives). This is usually done under granite or steel millstones that resemble those used more than 1,000 years ago. The paste is then spread onto thin mats, which are stacked and placed into a machine press. As the press applies several hundred pounds of pressure, oil and water seep out of the mats and drip into collection vats. This process requires no heat—hence the term "first cold-pressed" olive oil.

A bit confused about the term "cold press," let alone "first," I contacted food-science columnist Robert L.Wolke, professor emeritus of chemistry at the University of Pittsburgh and author of *What Einstein Told His Cook: Kitchen Science Explained* (W.W. Norton & Company, 2005). He gave me the lowdown on cold-pressing semantics: "Cold pressed means that the olives or the press are not heated or treated with hot water. The maximum allowed temperature for extra virgin oil is 25°C or 77°F. Heat would give a higher yield of oil during the pressing, but would compromise the quality and flavor. But that 'cold' or unheated pressing is the only pressing. The olives are virtually never pressed a second time at higher pressure, which would just squeeze bitter juices out of the pits. Instead, the remaining oil is coaxed out with hot water or an organic solvent. That oil, however, is a lower quality and cannot be labeled 'extra virgin.' Still, producers like to claim 'first pressing' for their extra virgin oils. It just sounds impressive."

Other methods, I learned, are also sometimes used to extract oil from olives. One is centrifugation. "A centrifuge spins materials around rapidly, like the spin cycle on a washing machine," explains Wolke. "After the pressing, it separates oil from the watery juices." However, mechanical pressing is the most popular way.

After pressing, the oil is then left to settle, and any vegetable water is removed by centrifuge machines. When the olive oil is created, it is set aside to be evaluated for its quality and categorized. And there are more terms to decode in the world of olive oil.

GRADES OF OLIVE OIL

Ever wonder what the differences are between "extra virgin," "virgin," and "pure" olive oils? Here's the real deal.

Extra virgin: Extracted from the highest-quality olives. It must have less than 1 percent natural acidity. Its "fruity" flavor is intense and great in salads.

Virgin: Processed mechanically (using pressure) and without heat, which changes the oil's acidity to 1 to 5 percent. It's recommended for use in salad dressings and marinades.

Pure: A mix of refined olive oil (treated with steam and chemicals) and virgin oils. Its acidity ranges from 3 to 4 percent. Less costly, it's most often used in cooking.

Extracted and refined: Made from whole cull olives and extracted during a second pressing with a chemical solvent; virgin oil is added for flavor.

Pomace: Made by a chemical extraction of the residue left over after the crushing and second pressing of the olives. It contains 5 to 10 percent acidity; virgin oil is added for flavor.

All-Natural Processing

Olive oil expert Dr. Deane confirms that extra virgin olive is one of the few oils that can be consumed and enjoyed without chemical processing. "Fresh pressed olive oil can be eaten immediately, and retains the natural flavors, vitamins, minerals, antioxidants, and other healthy products of the ripe olive fruit," he notes.

THE DA VINCI DECODED LABELS LEXICON

It's not uncommon to read words, including "blended olive oil" to "first cold press," on olive oil bottles and cans. Here is a quick glance at the meanings to help you decode what these olive oil terms really mean.

Terms to Know	Definition	The Real Deal
Blended olive oil	Combination of various olive types, regions, and countries	Grocery store brands are often blended
Imported from Italy	Gives the impression that the olives were grown in Italy	The fact is, the oil was bottled there
100 percent pure olive oil	A quality found in retail grocery stores	Better grades include "virgin" on the label
Made from refined olive oils	Hints that the essence is inside the bottle	In reality, the taste and acidity were chemically produced
Light olive oil	Insinuates a low fat content	The term points to a lighter color, not fewer calories or less fat
From hand-picked olives	Suggests that Mom and Pop gave the olives personal TLC	Vague about the harvest method—hands-on or tree-shaking
First cold press	Implies this is the number-one oil that came from the first press of the olives	The key word is "cold," because if heat is used, the olive oil's chemistry is changed

THE OLIVE CITY

Before I spread my wings and take you to meet olive experts worldwide and discover olive oils, I want to reiterate that I never knew that olives have been growing in California for centuries. Nor did I know that California's Corning, coined the Olive City, is home to the Bell Carter Olive Company, the world's largest ripe olive cannery. But while there are at least 300 varieties of olives grown from Oroville to Modesto in California, the Mission and Manzanillo are the most commonly used for olive oil.

FUN FACTS ABOUT CALIFORNIA RIPE OLIVES

You see them all the time. They're in many of your favorite foods and recipes—or maybe you like to eat them all by themselves. But how much do you know about California Ripe Olives? The California olive industry and California Ripe Olives provided some intriguing factoids:

Olives are a member of the fruit family.

Olives grow on trees and may have been first cultivated over 5,000 years ago in Syria and Crete.

In the 1700s, monks brought olives to Mexico and then to California by way of missions. The first cuttings were planted in 1769 at the San Diego Mission.

Commercial cultivation of California olives began in the late 1800s.

Today, anywhere from 80,000 to 106,000 tons of olives are produced in California each year.

About 70 to 80 percent of all ripe olives are grown in California's approximately 35,000 acres.

Olive trees bloom each year in May, and by mid-September, the olives are ready to be picked.

Olives, as they come from the tree, are too bitter to eat, so they are cured.

Four main varieties of olives are grown in California:

Mission—originally cultivated by the Franciscan missions.

Manzanillo—the most prevalent.

Sevillano—the larger size.

Ascolano—the larger size.

California Ripe Olives grow in a variety of sizes: small, medium, large, extra large, jumbo, colossal, and super colossal.

Olive trees tend to alternate their yields, producing large crops one year and smaller crops the next.

Olives destined for canneries are picked when they are still green and then become Ripe Olives.

Black ripe olives are oxidized, during processing; they are never dyed.

Medical doctors, nutritionists, olive oil producers and manufacturers, chefs, and consumers are now learning what people during biblical times practiced. True, in past centuries it was not known exactly how or why olive oil had healing powers—but it did. It's clear as a bottle of freshly pressed olive oil that peasants to royalty knew that olive oil had versatile virtues, worked wonders, and was as good as gold.

Mediterranean Shrimp Kabob

❖ ❖ ❖

MARINADE

¼ cup olive oil

2 teaspoons grated lemon peel

¼ cup fresh lemon juice

1 teaspoon Greek seasoning

½ teaspoon oregano

½ teaspoon salt

KABOBS

¾ lb. large raw shrimp, shelled and deveined*

12 canned, extra small artichoke heart quarters

12 large, pitted Kalamata olives

2 tablespoons crumbled feta cheese, optional

Combine olive oil, lemon peel, lemon juice, Greek seasoning, oregano, and salt in large plastic food storage bag; shake to mix well. Add shrimp and seal; toss to coat. Marinate in refrigerator at least 4 hours or overnight, turning occasionally.

Heat grill to medium direct heat. Meanwhile, add artichoke heart pieces and olives to marinade; toss to coat. Thread shrimp, artichokes, and olives on four 12-inch to 14-inch skewers (or place in grill basket). Grill covered for 5 to 8 minutes or until shrimp are opaque, turning once or twice. Remove to serving platter; sprinkle with feta cheese, if desired.

*Variation: If desired, substitute 3 boneless, skinless chicken breast halves for shrimp. Cut chicken into 1½-inch pieces. Marinate and grill as directed for shrimp. Serves 4.

(*Source:* North American Olive Oil Association)

THE GOLDEN SECRETS TO REMEMBER

New research shows that olive oil, especially polyphenol-rich extra virgin olive oil, which is made from a variety of olives in the Mediterranean countries—as well as from other places around the globe—may help you to:

- ✓ Lower your risk of heart disease and cancer.
- ✓ Enhance your immune system.
- ✓ Prevent cancer.
- ✓ Stave off diabetes.
- ✓ Fight fat.
- ✓ Slow the aging process.
- ✓ Add years to your life.

Most important, the quality of olive oil matters for your health's sake. Natural, organic, and cold pressed are recommended by olive oil producers to medical doctors.

In this book, I will show you how using olive oil (and other popular healing cooking oils) is one of the best things you can do for yourself—and your health. But note, many people will not want to reap the benefits of olive oil by swallowing a tablespoon (or two) solo. While olive oil is great on salads, it also is a great seasoning for many foods. Olive oil has a vast number of uses in cooking, and I've included more than 75 recipes to help heal your body, mind, and spirit. And the versatile oil can do so much more.

But first, let's go way, way back into the past. Take a close-up look at why and how olive oil is one of the world's first—and most prized—natural medicines.

A Genesis of the Olive

🌿

The olive tree is surely the richest gift of
Heaven, I can scarcely expect bread.
                    —Thomas Jefferson[1]

My first real-life olive oil experience was when I was a simple, hearty, food-loving eight-year-old kid who loved different places and different people. Did I enjoy different foods? Not so much because my Westernized palate wasn't worldly. One rainy Christmas Eve, my parents took my older sister, Debbie, and me to a modest San Jose, California, red, two-story apartment complex we had lived at before moving to our fifties' *Father Knows Best*–type house in the suburbs.

At the old complex to visit former neighbors, I knocked on Florence's upstairs front door. A short, plump, elderly gray-haired Italian lady greeted us—damp and cold—with a hug and genuine smile. I liked her and her kitchen filled with sweet and savory smells. After all, she baked cookies and breads. I sipped hot cocoa topped with miniature marshmallows; I sat huddled up to the warm stove. The kitchen table was cluttered with dozens of cans and bottles of oils and fats.

Florence offered me a cookie from a tin box. I asked, "Which ones should I choose?" She answered, "The long cookies with almonds—biscotti." She told me the oblong-shaped biscuit, twice-baked, was from Italy. I dipped it into my cocoa; she put hers in black tea. The woman whispered while pointing to a dark colored bottle on the table, "Olive oil makes cookies moist." She added, "My secret ingredient." I believed her. She gave me the box filled with layers of different biscotti including gingersnap, Neapolitan, pumpkin, and spumoni. It was a memorable special gift.

The art of using olive oil for physical and mental well-being goes back 6,000 years. As early as 400 B.C., Hippocrates, "the father of medicine," used olive oil in over 60 therapeutic remedies to treat his patients. In the era of the Romans and Egyptians, olive oil was mixed with herbs for medicinal treatments. Olive oil has been more than just a food to the people of the Mediterranean—it has been a medicinal agent and antibiotic, and has even provided promises of vitality, strength, and much more. Century after century, people discovered that the golden liquid works wonders for health.[2]

Today, medical doctors, nutritionists, and researchers around the world continue to find more and more powerful uses for this universal oil. And history shows that people since biblical times have taken advantage not only of the internal benefits of olive oil, but of its external perks as well.

Olive oil's great power is timeless. The earliest historical record of olive oil appears to be when Homer, the legendary early Greek poet, called olive oil "liquid gold" in the famous work *The Odyssey*. In ancient Greece, athletes rubbed it from head to toe. Not only did the golden liquid illuminate alive and beautiful bodies, but it was also used on the dead bodies of saints and heroes in their tombs.

HEALING OILS IN BIBLICAL TIMES

The olive tree was praised as the most valuable and versatile tree during the biblical era. Oil is mentioned 191 times in the Bible; seven of these times refer to olive oil, but in 147 of the references to oil, olive oil can be inferred by the reader, according to the *Healing Oils of the Bible*'s author, David Stewart, Ph.D.[3]

He explains, "When olive oil was extracted in Biblical times, the whole fruit was crushed by a stone wheel (as at Gethsemane) or mashed by treading under foot (as in Micah 6:5). The broken olives were placed in special baskets where the oil was allowed to drain into vats or basins by the force of gravity. This could take a few hours or a day or two. In the Bible, the resulting product was called 'first oil,' 'beaten oil,' or 'fine oil.' (Numbers 28:5)"[4]

Adds Stewart, "In today's language we call this 'virgin oil.' The oil that drains in the first hour or so is called 'extra virgin,' while that which drains later is simply called 'virgin.'"[5]

One of the most unforgettable references to olive oil and its remarkable healing powers is in the parable of the Good Samaritan who tends to a beaten and robbed traveler. The cure-all for treating the down-and-out individual's wounds is simply with oil and wine.

Here are some other interesting biblical references to the olive leaf, fruit, and tree. These were gleaned from a variety of sources all leading to the Bible:

- "His branches shall spread, and his beauty shall be as the olive tree." (Hosea 14:6)
- "Mount of Olives—so called because of the olive trees that cover its sides, is a mountain ridge to the east of Jerusalem." (1 Kings 11:7; Ezek. 11:23; Zech. 14:4)

- "For the Lord thy God bringeth thee into a good land, a land of brooks of water, of fountains and depths that spring out of valleys and hills; a land of wheat, and barley, and vines, and fig trees, and pomegranates; a land of olive trees and honey." (Deuteronomy 8:7–9)

In many regions, it's believed that the news of the end of the great flood was delivered by a single dove carrying one green olive tree branch in its beak. Later, the vivid image of that dove with the olive branch became the symbol of peace around the world. A reference in the Bible states: "And the dove came in to him in the evening, and lo, in her mouth was an olive leaf plucked off. So Noah knew that the waters were abated from off the earth." (Genesis 8:11)

Not only has it been noted that Christian missionaries brought the olive tree with them for food as well as religious ceremonies, but olive oil was also believed to be the oil of choice to anoint the kings of the Greeks and the Jews.

While the people in biblical times may have been clueless as to why olive oil had healing powers, they considered it a valuable staple in meals and used it both in cooking and on the table.

Since that period, olive oil is no longer the stuff of folk medicine and old wives' tales. Modern science is proving that folk healers were right all along. Both then and now, the precious oil is touted for its versatile uses and healthful properties, for the total body, mind, and spirit.

And, of course, the olive tree—the source of the sacred olive—is not to be ignored. Roman mythology attributes the birth of healing olives to Hercules, who struck the ground and caused an olive tree to sprout.[6] But there's more . . .

ODE TO THE OLIVE TREE

The olive tree has a long, long history of proving its value to people around the world since biblical times. It is mentioned in both the Old Testament and Greek mythology. It's been noted as the symbol of wisdom and peace.

Remember Athena, the legendary goddess of Greece? While Roman mythology links the olive tree to Hercules, the sacred olive is also connected to the goddess Athena and Athens. As the legend goes, Zeus had decreed that the city should be given to the god who offered the most useful gift to the people. Poseidon gave them the horse. Athena struck the bare soil with her spear and caused an olive tree to spring up. The people were so happy with the olive that Zeus gave the city to Athena and named it Athens after her.[7]

In the past, olive trees were recognized as sturdy and priceless. Olive tree leaves, fruit, and oil have been touted for centuries for their variety of health virtues, from healing properties to antiaging benefits.

So where exactly does the variety of tree grow and what does it look like, anyhow? It is evergreen, native to the Mediterranean region but grown in tropical areas and warm climates. The hard, yellow wood of the gnarled trunk is covered by gray-green bark. The branches extend to a height of 25 feet or more.

The leathery olive leaves are elliptic, oblong, or lanceolate in shape. They are dark green on top and have silvery scales underneath. The fragrant white flowers grow in axillary panicles that are shorter than the leaves. The fruit is an oblong or nearly round drupe that is shiny black when ripe. The best part is, the life span of an olive tree can be more than 1,500 years.

OIL, GREEKS, AND ROMANS

The Greeks and Romans both share legends about olives and their creation by the gods. At the ancient Olympic Games, winners were awarded an olive tree branch. The Greeks believed that the life of the sacred tree was transmitted to the taker through the branch. Even more amazing, it's been said that the Greeks valued the golden liquid to such an extent that they allowed only virgin boys and girls to pick olives.[8]

In ancient Greece and Rome, olive oil was a respected commodity (as well as taxed) and carried by trading ships to all the Mediterranean countries. The concept that olive oil provides strength and youth made it a precious liquid to have and to hold. Aromatics (such as roses and sage) were added to olive oil to make ointments as well as fuel for lamps. In Greece, Rome, and Egypt, olive oil was infused with flowers and grasses to make both beauty aids and medicine.[9]

Therapeutic Oil Formula of the Four Thieves

In the Middle Ages, oil made its mark during the scourge of the bubonic plague, or "Black Death," of Europe. Robbers in the French town of Marseilles stole the belongings left behind by the people who fell victim to the outbreak.

The legend is that these robbers were spice traders and perfumers. To avoid the deadly plague, they put the magic of their essential oils (such as garlic, eucalyptus, lemon, rosemary, and sage) to work by washing themselves with the infection-fighting liquid. Later, the thieves' oil formula was used by priests and doctors who treated the ill.

The Roman Empire embraced the cultivation of olive groves. But when the Roman Empire fell, the olive groves died, although some trees continued to thrive in Tuscany. In A.D. 1100, olive groves sprouted again, and Tuscany became a well-known region for harvesting the olive tree. In fact, in 1400, Italy was ranked the number-one producer of olive oil on the globe.[10]

By the fifteenth century B.C., olive cultivation had extended from Crete, Greece, to Syria, Palestine, and Israel, and then to Turkey, Cyprus, and Egypt. Until 1500 B.C., it was in Greece, however, according to reports, where olive trees were most widespread. After the sixteenth century, olive trees were also found in Spain.[11]

In the eighteenth century, Franciscan missionaries carried the first olive trees to America. And then, in the nineteenth century, olive oil became a well-known commodity in the United States when Italian and Greek immigrants demanded the golden liquid to be imported from Europe. Once a European treasure, olive oil soon also became as good as gold to the chefs in the New World.[12]

OLIVE OIL MAKES A SPLASH IN AMERICA

In the 1950s (when I was born and during which time I often ate a meat-and-potatoes diet combined with TV dinners and fast food), Ancel Keys, an American nutritionist and epidemiologist, conducted his famous Seven Countries Study. Keys and his colleagues studied the diet and health of the people in five European countries and compared their data with the data collected in similar studies in the United States and Japan. The findings: People who ate less saturated fat had lower levels of cholesterol and less heart disease than people who ate a high-saturated-fat diet.

During the 1950s, people, such as the Cretes in Greece, who followed a traditional Mediterranean diet and lifestyle—

including using olive oil (a monounsaturated fat)—had lower cholesterol levels and lower rates of heart disease. It was believed that a diet chock-full of fresh vegetables, seasonal fruits, whole grains, fish, meats, and olive oil—like what was eaten in the Mediterranean basin—was a healthful, heart-healthy plan.

As time passed, in the 1950s and '60s, scientists started to study different types of fat—including polyunsaturated fats, which seemed to reduce cholesterol levels better than monounsaturated fats. This, in turn, resulted in praising Crisco (originated in the early twentieth century), corn oil, and margarine (oleo), which I remember sitting in our refrigerator along with plenty of frozen and processed foods, while shunning butter as a "bad" fat and calling olive oil "neutral."

Later, in the 1970s and '80s, when I was a vegan hippie and penniless graduate student, health-conscious people, like me, said so long to butter and margarine and began to use polyunsaturated vegetable oils in rice and vegetable dishes. At this time, I had no clue that researchers were busy at work labeling high-density lipoproteins (HDL) as "good" cholesterol and low-density lipoproteins (LDL) as "bad" cholesterol in our bodies. I was just a 20-something kid. What did I know?

Then, we were told that saturated fat raised the "bad" cholesterol and lowered the "good" cholesterol, but that vegetable oils (such as corn, safflower, soybean and margarine), while they lowered the "bad" LDL cholesterol, could also lower the "good" HDL cholesterol. So, dazed and confused, before I received my master's degree in May 1990, the word was out to use polyunsaturated vegetable fats sparingly, to stay clear of saturated animal fats, and to embrace monounsaturated fats like olive oil.

In 1990, when I was out of graduate school, the scientific

jury was in. Research had shown that, rather than clog our arteries with saturated and polyunsaturated fats, we should turn to monounsaturated fats, which are rich in disease-fighting antioxidants.

Today, in the twenty-first century, olive oil (especially extra virgin olive oil) continues to gain praise worldwide for its vitamin E, phenol compounds, phytoestrogens, carotenoids, chlorophyll, and other good-for-you components. It plays a role in healthful cuisines—all types—in both restaurants and homes in the United States, as well as worldwide.

OTHER PAST MEDICAL USES OF OLIVE OIL

Historical Olive Oil

User	Method	Ailment
Biblical priests	Olive oil paired with aromatics	To treat leprosy
Goddess Athena	Olive oil	To use as medicine
Greek athletes	Olive oil	To cleanse their bodies
Greeks, Egyptians, Romans	Infused olive tree flowers with grass or essential oils	To use as ointment for cuts, sores, bleeding wounds, bruises, and other injuries
Homer	Olive oil	Called it "liquid gold"

OTHER PAST MEDICAL USES OF OLIVE OIL (*cont.*)

Historical Olive Oil

User	Method	Ailment
Hippocrates	Mixture of olive oil and leaves	To treat boils, cholera, inflammation of gums, muscle pain, nausea, and ulcers
Italians	Olive oil	To increase strength and youthful vitality
Christopher Columbus	Olive oil	Provided it to his exploring team

OLIVE OIL MILESTONES

Year	What Happened	What It Did
1500s	Olive trees were part of the landscape in Spain	Spain ended up being the number-one olive oil producer
1600s	First olive press in the world was created on the island of Crete[13]	This paved the way for olive oil to be made and distributed
1800s	Olive oil made its debut in America	Olive oil was soon used by American cooks

OLIVE OIL MILESTONES (cont.)

Year	What Happened	What It Did
1950s	Professor Ancel Keys, an American scientist, did research work to link the people of the Greek island of Crete to the Mediterranean diet	His Seven Countries Study showed that a diet low in saturated fat and high in monounsaturated and polyunsaturated fats may be the key to the Cretes' low rate of heart disease and increased longevity
1950s–1960s	Polyunsaturated fats were touted, saturated fats were shunned	This raised awareness about the dietary fat–health connection
1970s–1980s	HDL and LDL cholesterol was studied	"Bad" dietary fats such as polyunsaturated and saturated fats were linked to lowering "good" cholesterol and increasing "bad" cholesterol
1975	*How to Eat Well and Stay Well the Mediterranean Way* by Dr. Ancel Keys and Margaret Keys was published	It popularized the heart-healthy diet
1983	*Feast of the Olive* by Maggie Blythe Klein was published	It taught how to cook with olives and olive oil

OLIVE OIL MILESTONES (*cont.*)

Year	What Happened	What It Did
1988	Anne Dolamore's *Essential Olive Oil Companion* was published	It allowed readers to appreciate not only the olive but also its oil
1980s	Consumers were told to use monounsaturated fats such as olive oil, to use small amounts of polyunsaturated fats, and to stay clear of saturated fats	This allowed people to lower their risk of heart disease by eating a heart-healthy diet
1990s	American scientists published articles on the Mediterranean diet	The articles linked lowered incidences of health problems with eating fresh vegetables, fruits, grains, fish, meats, and olive oil
1995	*Enter the Zone* by Barry Sears, Ph.D. was published	It praised "good" monounsaturated fats such as olive oil and olives
Early 2000s	Olive oil expands in popularity	Olive oil begins to play a role around the globe in diet, health, beauty, household use, and more

OLIVE OIL MILESTONES (cont.)

Year	What Happened	What It Did
2015	Olive oil paired with other oils and saturated fats for cooking, baking, and cosmetic use in moderation boasts health perks	Healing olive oil leads the pack of oils, but other cooking oils and fats are getting recognition

Tender Focaccia

❖ ❖ ❖

This focaccia, with a crumb softened by the addition of both potato flour and dry milk, is ideal for slicing and turning into sandwiches.

2 cups (16 ounces)
 boiling water
3¾ cups (16 ounces)
 unbleached all-purpose
 flour
2½ teaspoons instant yeast
¼ cup (1½ ounces) potato
 flour, or ⅓ cup (¾
 ounce) potato flakes
¼ cup (1¼ ounces) nonfat
 dry milk

1½ teaspoons salt
2 tablespoons (⅞ ounce)
 olive oil, plus 2 to 3
 tablespoons to grease
 the pan and the surface
 of the dough
¼ to ½ teaspoon kosher
 salt, sea salt, or fleur de
 sel, for topping
Few sprigs of fresh herb

Put the boiling water and 2 cups of the all-purpose flour in a large bowl and beat for several minutes to develop a smooth batter. If you have the time, add ⅛ teaspoon yeast once the batter has cooled to lukewarm and set the sponge aside for several hours or overnight; this helps develop flavor in the finished loaf, as well as the soft interior texture.

Whisk the potato flour or potato flakes with the remaining flour, dry milk, yeast, and salt. Add this to the batter a little at a time, while continuing to beat. Add 2 tablespoons of olive oil. Beat, by hand with a large spoon or with the paddle attachment of a mixer set at medium speed, for 8 to 10 minutes, changing to a dough hook when the dough begins to hold together.

After the dough has become smooth and shiny, put it in an oiled bowl, cover it with a damp towel or plastic wrap, and let it rise for 30 minutes. The dough should have increased by about one-third and be puffy-looking. Don't punch down the dough, but rather pull the sides of the dough up and over in a folding motion. Do this several times to release some of the gas, then let the dough rise for another 30 minutes.

Drizzle 2 tablespoons of olive oil into a 12- or 14-inch round pan or 1 tablespoon olive oil into each of two 8-inch round pans. Place the dough in the oiled pan(s), gently stretching it to fit. Let the dough rest for 30 minutes, then stretch it out a little more. At this point, you may refrigerate the dough in the pan(s), tightly covered, for up to 24 hours.

Preheat the oven to 400°. Just before baking the focaccia, dimple it with your fingers, brush it with a little olive oil, and sprinkle it with coarse kosher or sea salt or a few sprigs of fresh herb. Bake the focaccia for 25 to 30 minutes, until it's deep brown all over. Remove it from the pan(s) and cool it for 15 minutes before eating. Serve with flavored olive oil or split for sandwiches. Two 8-inch round or one 12- or 14-inch round focaccia. 12 servings.

(*Source: The King Arthur Flour Baker's Companion: All-Purpose Baking Cookbook*)

THE GOLDEN SECRETS TO REMEMBER

As you can see, liquid gold has been touted for good reason—in America and around the world—as a valuable healing medicine. Olive oil lovers past and present believe that healing oils—olive oil and other oils, too—add years to your life by:

- ✓ Acting as a medicinal agent—solo or teamed with herbs—to fight dozens of health ailments and diseases.
- ✓ Fighting the infection of wounds.
- ✓ Soothing inflammation, muscle pain, and other medical disorders.
- ✓ Providing a versatile staple in meals.
- ✓ Offering a symbol of peace worldwide.
- ✓ Enhancing energy and stamina.
- ✓ Acting as a heart-healthy food in the Mediterranean diet.

No doubt, olive oil, since biblical times, has had an amazing track record of powerful health benefits. And it's continued to hold up its good name, as well as create a mighty buzz around the world. In Part 2, "Olive Oil," you'll discover some amazing facts and meet intriguing people from the Mediterranean world. Now it's time to get the lowdown on one of the world's most popular kinds of oil—olive oil—in the twentieth and twenty-first centuries.

PART 2

OLIVE OIL

A Historical Testimony

Wash him in the stream of the river, Anoint him
with immortal oil, Put him on the divine tunic.
                                        —Homer[1]

My second encounter with olive oil was when I was a pre-teen and picky eater who had a thing for real butter, the kind served in fancy restaurants—not oil. My best girlfriend's mom, a woman who watched Julia Child on television, took us to the beach on Wednesdays because that was her day off.

She was an okay lady, but I didn't like her lunches. She put sautéed onions and vegetable oil on everything from meat loaf to salami sandwiches. Olive trees prefer coastal regions; maybe she knew that. But I was just a kid, not a tree. Sitting in the damp fog with a blanket wrapped around me, I told her, "I don't like to eat on the sand. The wind makes the bread and oil gritty."

One sunny, warm day after I didn't eat her stupid sandwiches, she asked me what kind of foods I liked to eat. I told her, "I love real butter on French bread." I forgot to tell her I didn't like oil on sandwiches. The next week I was happy with the cheese, butter, and sourdough bread she brought in the picnic basket. But as time passed, my distaste for olive oil drizzled on veggie and cheese sandwiches changed.

Olive oil was healthy in the twentieth century, and it is healthy in the twenty-first century, too. While its uses are infinite—both inside and outside the body—its healing powers are due to its healthful ingredients. And now, research shows promising benefits of the nutrients in olive oil (which may be missing from our daily food intake thanks to processed foods) more than ever before. But these new findings would not be surprising to the folks who have touted olive oil through the decades.

OLIVE OIL PIONEERS IN THE TWENTIETH CENTURY

Born in 1915, Joseph Sciabica was an olive oil maker since 1936. His father, Nicola, and he began with the grass-roots of olive oil production, which he learned in Sicily, Italy, as a young man.

In Waterbury, Connecticut, in the 1940s, it was common for Joseph to deliver a load of wine grapes and olive oil to an Italian family in the city. In fact, Nick Sciabica & Sons sold olive oil directly to Italian families from 1936 to 1968.

The late Joseph, who resided in Modesto, California, for decades, lived a long life into his nineties, while he enjoyed scores of olive trees and the fruit they gave to his business and family. He and his wife, Gemma, have had passed their knowledge on to both their sons, Daniel and Nick, and their grandson Jonathan. These days, Nick Sciabica & Sons makes 100 percent extra virgin natural cold-pressed olive oil.

Gemma Sanita Sciabica, a charming Italian woman in her eighties, also from Connecticut, was married to Joseph for more than half a century. She is a nutrition-savvy cook who has been creating healthful Italian-based recipes for years. Her cookbooks, such as *Cooking with California Olive Oil: Recipes from the Heart for the Heart,* are filled with heart-healthy recipes from the old Mediterranean world. But there are other olive growers in California, too, who have helped spread the healthful oil worldwide.

In the 1990s, once olive oil was embraced by America for its health benefits, California jumped on the Mediterranean bandwagon. "Wineries in Napa and Sonoma began to plant a few olives as an adjunct to their main business. The first grower to import Italian olives was Ridgely Evers of Healdsburg in 1990. He was followed by Nan McEvoy and Roberto Zecca, owners of Frantoio Restaurant," writes Charles Quest-Ritson in his book *Olive Oil* (DK Publishing, 2006).[2]

While I did not get to meet Zecca face to face, I did talk with him briefly on the telephone. Better still, I visited his unique and impressive restaurant. I knew, however, that Zecca has a place in the olive oil world, both in Italy and in Mill Valley, California.

As the story goes, in 1989, the retired banker and his wife, Christina, decided to relocate to the hills of Greve in Chianti. They bought a *Castellare*, which is a castle-villa. They began to make extra virgin olive oil from the grove of olive trees surrounding their home. At first, they made the healthy oil for their personal use, and then they began to sell it to local markets.

A few years later, the couple came to Northern California and opened a one-of-a-kind restaurant that included a *frantoio,* or olive press. In the fall of 1995, the Frantoio Olive Oil Co. produced its first crush. And these days, Zecca offers an olive oil tagged Select Sevillano, as well as provides a popular place to enjoy great Italian cuisine and view the making of healthy extra virgin olive oil.

A Toast to the Green Olive and Martini

Before California olive oil pioneers made their mark in the Golden State, another pioneer, of sorts, brought the world the green olive in a dry martini. I prefer the story linking the concoction to a gold miner in Martinez, in Northern California. Back in the mid-nineteenth century, the miner understandably wanted to celebrate his gold strike. At a bar, he asked for a special drink made with gin and vermouth and topped with bitters and a maraschino cherry. The drink was coined the "martini," in respect for the town Martinez. Decades later, someone else opted to use a green olive instead of a cherry. And today, some people use different garnishes, from a slice of lemon peel to two green olives rich in monounsaturated fat.

MR. CHOLESTEROL—DR. ANCEL KEYS

Ancel Keys, Ph.D., who was born in 1904 and lived nearly 100 years, is the man who focused on one of America's biggest problems, past and present—heart disease. He is the man behind the Seven Countries Study. For several decades, he kept his eyes on 12,000 middle-aged men from Italy, the Greek Islands, Yugoslavia, the Netherlands, Finland, Japan, and the United States. His findings were that saturated fat (found in butter and cheese) was linked to high cholesterol and heart attacks. But things change. (Refer to Chapter 8, "More Healing Oils," to find out the latest scoop on butter—all types—and health.)

However, a Mediterranean diet based on fresh vegetables, fruit, bread, pasta—and the monounsaturated fat olive oil—showed that high cholesterol and heart attacks were not part of the picture. He made the diet–heart disease connection. In fact, in the 1950s, when Keys visited Greece to find out why Cretes lived longer than the people of other cultures, he was astonished by how much olive oil these people used on their salads.

Dr. Keys is known for two diets he popularized. He created balanced meals for soldiers that were called "K rations." Later on, the health-conscious doctor and his wife, Margaret, made the Mediterranean diet known through two books, *Eat Well and Stay Well* (Doubleday, 1959) and *How to Eat Well and Stay Well the Mediterranean Way* (Doubleday, 1975).

OLIVE OYL LINKS TO OIL

In the 1950s and '60s, while serious doctors were praising the powers of olive oil, kids and their parents watched the popular *Popeye* cartoons, which also were linked to olive oil, but in a humorous way that made its impression on a large audience, too.

Elzie Segar created Olive Oyl for his comic strip, "Thimble Theater," back in 1919. The tall, thin cartoon character with black hair is named after olive oil. Segar's newspaper comics also feature a variety of Olive Oyl's relatives, tagged after other oils, such as her brother, Castor Oyl, and their mother, Nan Oyl (after banana oil).

Olive Oyl gained popularity in the animated television cartoons, where she is Popeye's girlfriend. Bluto (also known as the bully Brutus) is Popeye's competition for Olive's attention, but the sailor always eats his spinach and rescues the damsel in distress, who ironically has a baby named Swee' Pea.

CONTEMPORARY DOCTORS: THE OLIVE OIL ADVOCATES

In 1996, I interviewed best-selling author Dr. Barry Sears, who had written the popular book *Enter the Zone* (Harper-Collins, 1995). Working on a weight-loss-diet story for *Woman's World* magazine, I was a bit surprised when the doctor told me fat was part of his dietary plan, since I was writing about low-fat and fat-free foods. But today, I understand that he was ahead of his time.

More than 10 years ago, he wrote in his book that while saturated fats should be kept to a minimum, there are also "good" fats. He put it this way: "Most of the good fats are monounsaturated fats—those found in olive oil, canola oil, olives, macadamia nuts, and avocados (and, of course, guacamole). (A diet rich in monounsaturated fats is sometimes called a Mediterranean diet or the "Medi-diet.")

In a nutshell, he advised staying clear of "bad" fats such as saturated fats (found in animal protein sources and whole-fat dairy products), and getting most of your daily fat from "good," monounsaturated fat.

While the Zone diet is a high-protein diet, Dr. Sears is still an advocate of "good" fats rich in monounsaturated fat.

On the flip side, Jan McBarron, M.D., a Columbus, Georgia, weight-loss specialist that I have interviewed several times throughout the years, has put protein on the side. She includes olive oil (like Dr. Sears recommends), but she shed unwanted pounds herself by following a Mediterranean-type diet and lifestyle. She eats heartily early in the day, focuses on complex carbohydrates, keeps protein intake moderate, has small snacks throughout the day, and gets moderate exercise.

Dr. McBarron's meal plan is based on complex carbohydrates. A diet of 70 percent complex carbs—vegetables, fruits, pasta, rice, bread, lentils, peas, and beans—provides more energy than one full of protein-rich foods, so you'll burn more fat, she says. "Complex carbohydrates also stimulate the production of serotonin, a brain chemical that can ease stress that leads to overeating." And speaking of food . . .

Dr. McBarron adds, "I'm married to an Italian. He grew up having pasta seven days a week. We always have pasta on the table. I'll have it four to five times a week. My husband is extremely healthy. He was raised on a healthy diet. When I met him I always did the salad dressing on the side because I was trying to watch my weight. And he always had oil and vinegar. I thought, 'Oh, that sounds terrible.' I don't even have salad dressing in my house anymore—it's always oil and vinegar for the taste and nutrients in it." And olive oil is more than a good-for-you food. It's a sacred oil to some people.

OLIVE OIL IN RELIGION

Before I take you back into the world of nutrition and your kitchen, I can't ignore the fact that olive oil is dished up in religion and folk magic. It is common knowledge that olive oil has been used for centuries by Christians as well as the ancient Hebrews. The sacred oil was also used for anointing the kings of the Kingdom of Israel and in religious ceremonies of the ancient Minoans.

"During baptism in the Christian church, holy oil, which is often olive oil, may be used for anointment. At the Chrism mass, olive oil blessed by the bishop, 'chrism,' is used in the ceremony," explains John Deane, M.D.

As a Catholic woman, religion and holy oil brings back fond childhood memories of learning the seven sacraments and playing a role in some of them—which included using olive oil. In fact, before 1970, olive oil was used in four of the seven sacraments—Baptism, Confirmation, Holy Orders, and Anointing of the Sick. In 1970, holy oils were allowed to come from any plant, not just olives. But olive oil is still used in most dioceses, and the only reason it is not used is that it isn't available.

Baptism: I know firsthand that the Catholic and Orthodox Churches use olive oil for the Oil of Catechumen (used to bless and strengthen those preparing for Baptism). At Saint Joseph's Church in San Jose, California, I was baptized on the sixteenth of November 1952 according to the Rite of the Roman Catholic Church. As an infant, I had the sign of the cross made on my forehead with the holy oil.

Anointing of the Sick: I recall when I was 10 years old, our neighbor, Dale, was suffering with many illnesses. She was wheelchair-bound and in pain from the effects of polio. She, like my family, was Catholic. My mom told me that a priest from our parish paid her a home visit to bless her. These days, I know that this sacrament is called "Anointing of the Sick." Again, the blessed olive oil was used in a sign of the cross on both her forehead and hands.

Confirmation: As a teenager, I was confirmed at Saint Frances Cabrini's Church in San Jose, California. My confirmation name was Theresa, chosen by me. Again, I was anointed by a bishop who used the sign of the cross on my forehead during the ceremony. Today, I still feel bonded to the Catholic Church. However, I am open-minded and don't judge other religions around the world.

It's Time to Eat Pray Love

One of my favorite chick flicks is *Eat Pray Love*. The protagonist, Liz, played by actor Julia Roberts, enjoys a food fest that would make Ernest Hemingway blush. The indulgences take place in Rome but tend to make me hungry in the Sierra. In one scene, Liz announces she is "having a relationship" with her pizza napoletana (the scene was shot at L'Antica Pizzeria da Michele in Naples). And it was difficult not to call the pizza guy.

Not to forget the figs and ham when Liz walks through the streets of Rome. The food adventurer passes a woman cutting into a plate of fresh figs and Parma ham—almost a spellbinding ritual that made me want to book a flight abroad ASAP. And, of course, when Liz orders and savors each bite of the spaghetti all'amatriciana, a simple dish, including chili peppers, onions, pancetta, and olive oil, she makes it look like a meal fit for a princess or prince (images of the romantic scene of *Lady and the Tramp* sharing pasta come to mind).

Another fine scene for foodies with health on the brain, like me, is when Liz dines alone and prepares egg, asparagus, potato, and ham salad. When she drizzles olive oil on the food, it lured me to my kitchen pantry to make a meal (like a Stepford wife in a trance, I re-created the scene). Other food events, like the Thanksgiving dinner with good food and good people, and Liz ordering an array of dishes (in a foreign language she had mastered) for a group of dear Italian friends, are to be cherished.

Today, I aspire to make my dishes stand out in presentation like the foods viewed in *Eat Pray Love*. But in yesteryear as a tomboy, I flunked home economics in junior high. Worse, my mother didn't like me creating dishes in the kitchen. I didn't follow directions. I always modified cookbook recipes. But today, for the health and flavor of it, I am a fearless spiritual warrior in the kitchen. Cooking, baking, and dining can be a rebellious adventure each and every time for me, much like Liz embarking on food trips in Rome.

A Taste of Mediterranean Edibles

Here, take a close-up look at a few of my favorite Italian-style recipes I've created and dished up for myself, a woman from the San Francisco Bay Area living in the Sierra for more than a decade. I escape into the world of olive oil and use a touch of Mediterranean flair to my life without whisking off to Rome.

Chicken Cacciatore with Oils

❖ ❖ ❖

Enter chicken cacciatore (cacciatore means "hunter" in Italian). It's a complete meal made "hunter-style" with tomatoes, onions, herbs, bell pepper, and chicken. You can bake it or make it in a skillet on the stovetop. A common recipe calls for olive oil, a variety of chicken parts, wine, and tomatoes.

This recipe is adapted from my mother's chicken cacciatore. My version is like her tasty and memorable dish, sort of. But she used canned tomatoes (I do not like canned or frozen foods except for all-natural ice cream), a whole chicken, spices in cans, and white pasta—ingredients used in the twentieth century. Also, the dish would simmer for hours, unlike my meal with fresh stuff.

As a twenty-first-century post-hippie health nut, I put in the oil, leave out the wine, turn to skinless chicken breasts, and embrace fresh Roma tomatoes. I cook the meal faster rather than slower to save the nutrients of the vegetables. No Crock Pot for this one. And, of course, I use organic ingredients and whole grain pasta. (In the 1980s, pasta grew in popularity; it's still a popular staple teamed with olive oil in my diet repertoire.) A hearty stew like this is comfort food on cool autumn days. When I cook chicken cacciatore, it brings back a sense of security and warmth from my home in the suburbs. The aroma of garlic, onions, and veggies lingers in my home each time with this recipe of mine, a timeless favorite.

1 tablespoon each of olive oil and European-style butter
2 boneless, skinless chicken breasts
Pepper, to taste
½ cup red onion, chopped
1 garlic clove, minced

½ cup red bell pepper, chopped
4 Roma tomatoes, chopped
4 organic basil leaves
1 24-ounce jar of organic roasted pasta sauce with olive oil
2 cups whole wheat rotini, cooked

On medium heat, heat oil and butter in large skillet on stovetop. Add chicken (rinsed with water), sprinkle with pepper, cook about 5–6 minutes, and flip over for another 5 minutes. Place on plate.

In another large skillet, add red onion, garlic, red bell pepper, tomatoes, basil leaves, and pasta sauce. Stir for several minutes. Add chicken breasts. Cover and simmer on low-medium heat for about 10–15 minutes; turn to simmer for another 15 minutes or until chicken is tender and cooked.

Tip: If sauce is too thick, add a bit of water. Serve on top of whole grain pasta (follow the cooking instructions on the package) served with warm French bread dipped in garlic or basil olive oil and a tossed green salad. Serves 2–4 (depending on the size of the chicken breasts) with leftovers. (Note: All-natural store-bought sauces are doable, but to lose sodium to trans fats, make your own with fresh tomatoes, herbs, and spices.)

Sweet Potato Oven Fries

❖ ❖ ❖

Ah, the sound of sizzling taters in the oven is worth the time it takes to make them. Sure, I could have ordered this at a local restaurant or used store-bought frozen fries, but fixing it at home with rosemary olive oil paired with rich European-style butter for extra flavor is sublime. Munching hot, crispy fries works like a lucky rabbit's foot charm for me. This is an easy fail-proof recipe I put to work, time after time.

Two sweet potatoes, washed
2–3 tablespoons rosemary
*   olive oil*
1 tablespoon European-
*   style butter*

Sea salt and pepper to taste
2 tablespoons onion, diced
Malt vinegar and ketchup
*   for drizzling*

Preheat oven to 400°. Soak potatoes in hot water for about 5 minutes (this helps to make the fries crispier). Cut into thick slices with skins on. Place in pan and drizzle oil and butter on top. Sprinkle salt, pepper, and onion on top of potatoes. Put in oven. Turn mixture a few times to make sure potatoes get cooked evenly. Bake for about 30 minutes until golden brown. Drizzle with malt vinegar and ketchup to taste. Serves 2.

Fudgy Coconut Oil Brownies

❖ ❖ ❖

Welcome to fudgy brownies with both olive oil and coconut oil. Also, dark chocolate and nuts are part of this bar. This is a classic recipe, but with my own healing-oils spin of semi-homemade (the brownie mix nutrition label reads no trans fats). But note, these bars are good, so if you want to stave off a "muffin top" as noted in *Eat Pray Love*, savor one, not a whole batch like I did.

*¼ cup and 2 teaspoons
   extra virgin olive oil*
¼ cup coconut oil
2 organic brown eggs
¼ cup water
*1 package store-bought pre-
   mium dark chocolate
   brownie mix*

*¼ cup whole-wheat flour (at
   high altitude)*
½ cup dark chocolate chips
½ cup almonds, sliced
*1 cup sweetened coconut,
   shredded*

In a large bowl, combine oil, beaten eggs, and water. Add brownie mix and flour; stir till smooth. Fold in chocolate chips and almonds. Lightly grease (with extra virgin olive oil) an 8-inch-by-8-inch glass square dish; pour and spread brownie mixture. Bake at 325° for about 40 minutes. While warm from the oven, sprinkle top with shredded coconut. Makes about 12 brownies.

Italian Wedding Soup

❖ ❖ ❖

2 to 3 pounds of chicken
1 cup onion, chopped
2 cups celery, chopped
4 garlic cloves, minced
Sea salt and pepper to taste
½ cup parsley and/or basil
    chopped
3 to 4 quarts water
½ pound ground meat of
    your choice
1 egg

¼ cup Romano cheese
    grated
½ cup bread crumbs
¼ cup parsley, chopped
1 garlic clove
⅓ cup Marsala Olive Oil
1 head escarole, washed,
    chopped
½ cup orzo pasta (or any
    small pastina)

Boil, in a covered pot, chicken, onion, celery, garlic, salt, pepper, parsley, and water until chicken is tender; cool. Remove skin and bones; then chop meat and set aside. Strain broth and remove fat off top. Put aside.

Mix ground meat, egg, Romano cheese, bread crumbs, ¼ cup parsley, and garlic. Roll into balls. In large skillet, heat olive oil. Sauté balls on all sides until browned. Steam escarole until tender. Bring broth to a boil. Add chicken, escarole, meatballs, and orzo, then cook until tender. Serves 6.

(*Source: Cooking with California Olive Oil: Treasured Family Recipes* by Gemma Sanita Sciabica)

These days, while people use olive oil for religion, food, medicine, cosmetics, home cures, and lamps, there is an enormous supply of remarkable olive trees. But I have discovered that nobody knows for sure how many olive trees exist on Earth. According to the North American Olive Oil

Association, there are now more than 800 million olive trees planted worldwide. Paul Vossen of the University of California Cooperative Extension in Sonoma County, who studies the olive oil industry and educates its farmers, told me there are more than 24 million acres full of olive trees around the globe. The number of olive varieties, he adds, is around 2,500 to 3,000.

While people are putting olive oil to work in a variety of ways, there are also a number of powerful components that deserve due credit. In the next chapter, I'll show you what research has revealed about olive oil and its supernutrients—which are missing more and more from the diet here in America, in the Mediterranean basin, and worldwide.

THE GOLDEN SECRETS TO REMEMBER

✓ Extra virgin olive oil, which is polyphenol-rich, was made and sold in the early 1900s by olive oil pioneers on the East Coast who helped bring this liquid gold to the West Coast of America.
✓ Olive "oyl" and spinach—two healthy foods—were introduced in the early twentieth century in cartoons; and in the nineteenth century, the green olive made its debut in a popular alcoholic mixed drink.
✓ Olive oil has been used in religion for centuries—and in the twentieth century, the blessed oil was used as the main ingredient in four sacraments of the Catholic religion, and in other religions, too.

4

Where Are the Secret Ingredients?

*The grape and the olive are among the priceless
benefactions of the soil, and were destined, each
in its way, to promote the welfare of man.*
                                   —George Ellwanger[1]

Olive oil was sketchy to me as a child; but I remember how
liquid gold played a role in my early twenties. I hitched and
hiked through America in the winter with a knapsack, sleeping bag, and my black Labrador retriever, Stonefox. Like an
olive tree, we were tough and versatile. One afternoon, stranded
in a Wyoming blizzard, standing on a freeway ramp, I wasn't
dressed for freezing temperatures; my canine companion didn't
have a double dense coat like snow dogs. I spent my last three
dollars on hideous-looking yellow gloves to warm my chapped,
red hands (that could have benefited from soothing olive
oil). My best friend whined; his foot pads were red and cold.

After eternity, a diesel truck stopped. We were rescued by a truck driver and traveled through my first whiteout.

Later at a truck stop, we were treated to a meal. I ordered a gigantic chef's salad with plenty of Thousand Island dressing (on the side), French bread and butter, and black tea. I used olive oil and red wine vinegar (it came with the salad full of turkey, eggs, cheese, tomatoes, cucumbers, and greens). Although we survived the superstorm, a Nevada desert sandstorm, the Arizona heat, and the biblical rain in monsoon season (I prefer a Mediterranean climate like olive groves), colds hit me once too often. If I could go back in time (with my olive oil smarts), I would have carried EVOO and its counterpart vinegar in my pack for my diet and first aid. Here's why.

When you look at extra virgin olive oil's product label, it appears to be a health-minded person's ideal food: no trans fats, cholesterol, or sodium. But when I read the nutrition label, I didn't see vitamins or minerals. So, where are the powerful nutrients in olive oil, anyhow?

Dazed and confused, I went straight to the olive oil experts and obtained a nutritional breakdown of the golden liquid. The nutrition facts seem to be a bit different, and the measurements a bit bigger.

Supersize Olive Oil, Anyone?

100 grams (3½ ounces) of olive oil contains:

100 percent fat
1 milligram calcium
0.56 milligram iron
1 milligram potassium
2 milligrams sodium
0.3 milligram choline

0.1 milligram betaine
14.35 milligrams vitamin E
60.2 micrograms vitamin K
13.808 grams fatty acids, total saturated
72.961 grams fatty acids, total monounsaturated
10.523 grams fatty acids, total polyunsaturated
221 milligrams phytosterols

Apparently, more olive oil equals more nutrients. One cup contains about two times the amount of fat, calories, vitamins, and minerals.

(*Source:* National Nutrient Database for Standard Reference, 2006)

People who have written about olive oil claim that olive oil is chock-full of nutrients, minerals, and vitamins. True, the golden liquid does contain essential nutrients if you drink the stuff. The bottom line: Researchers know that quality extra virgin olive oil contains disease-fighting polyphenols, as well as other nutrients that can be effective if teamed with the Mediterranean diet and lifestyle. In other words, it's not the olive oil by itself that can contain healing powers. Speaking of olive oil . . .

QUALITY COUNTS

Not all olive oil is nutrient-rich, natural, organic, extra virgin olive oil made using the cold-pressed method. Some producers slow down the process or use heat so that the oil will taste better and can be preserved longer.

The fact is, the best olive oils are made from polyphenol-rich olives and cold-pressed within 24 to 48 hours after harvesting. This is the ideal way.

Olive oil contains the same important nutrients as olives—fat, calcium, and vitamins E and K—plus it contains other nutritional components.

So, What's in an Olive, Anyhow?

Three-and-one-half ounces of olives contains:

163 calories
70.8 percent water
1.2 grams protein
18.6 grams fat
1.7 grams fiber
79 milligrams calcium
200 international units vitamin A
0.01 milligram vitamin B_1
0.18 milligram vitamin B_2
0.1 milligram vitamin B_3
3 milligrams vitamin C
2.3 international units vitamin E

(*Source:* John Deane, M.D.)

SIX SUPER HEALTH-PROMOTING OLIVE OIL COMPONENTS

1 **Essential Fatty Acids:** Oleic acid is monounsaturated and makes up 55 to 85 percent of olive oil. Linoleic is polyunsaturated and makes up about 9 percent. Linolenic, which is polyunsaturated, makes up 0 to 1.5 percent. These types of fats, unlike trans fats, are heart healthy and much more.

Olive oil has no trans fatty acid. That's right; it has no unhealthy artery-clogging trans fats. It isn't a trans fatty acid because it hasn't been partially hydrogenated in a factory to make it solid at room temperature, like margarine.

Both omega-3 and omega-6 fatty acids also are in olive oil. Omega-3 fatty acids are important in preventing heart disease and are high in oily fish, such as salmon, and flaxseed oil. The jury is still out about how much omega-3 versus omega-6 you should incorporate into your daily diet.

Foods rich in essential fatty acids include fish, olive oils, fish oils and flaxseed oils. Team the olive oil with fish in our Simple Salmon* dish, and you'll get both "good" fats and good taste, too.

2 **Antioxidants:** Like essential fatty acids, the polyphenols in olive oil are good for your body from head to toe. Natural antioxidants have been scientifically proven to have a variety of health benefits, from healing sunburn to lowering cholesterol, blood pressure, and the risk of heart disease. There are as many as 5 milligrams of antioxidant polyphenols in every 10 grams of olive oil, according to Dr. Deane.

Vitamin E, for one, is a natural antioxidant in olive oil. One tablespoon provides 8 percent of the RDA for vitamin E. Research shows that people who eat antioxidant-rich foods such as vegetable oils, fruits, vegetables, grains, and nuts lower their risk of getting heart disease and cancer.

You can get antioxidants by eating antioxidant-rich foods such as vegetables and vitamin-E-rich olive oil. Just whip up a batch of our Sesame-Almond Vegetable Sauté,* and enjoy.

*Recipes found in Chapters 13 and 19.

3 **Calcium:** Olive oil also contains a trace of needed calcium. If your diet is deficient in calcium, your body will steal it from your bones. This, in turn, will weaken your skeleton and can lead to brittle bone disease.

Note these other important calcium facts:

- Ninety percent of the body's calcium is stored in the bones and teeth.
- One percent is found in the blood and tissues.
- Calcium is necessary for transmitting nerve impulses and regulating muscle contraction.
- The need for calcium starts in infancy and continues throughout life.

While olive oil may contain only a small amount of bone-boosting calcium, you can add it to calcium-rich dishes. Also, you don't have to stick with milk, yogurt, or cheese. Calcium is found in broccoli, green leafy vegetables, and tofu. Try our Broccoli Peanut Oil Stir-Fry* for that calcium fix you need.

4 **Iron:** Not only does your body need calcium, but it requires iron, too. As with calcium, olive oil contains just a small amount of iron, but you can certainly use it to make iron-rich dishes taste better. No, liver isn't the only source of iron. Remember Popeye? He got his iron from spinach. Go ahead—give our Cornish Game Hens with Orange Olive Oil* a try, and don't forget Olive "Oyl"—a must-have companion.

5 **Potassium:** Olive oil, again, contains just a small amount of potassium. But don't forget that olive oil can be teamed with vegetables, and that is where

you're going to get plenty of potassium. It's the potassium that helps energize you. Low potassium levels bring on fatigue. Often, people who suffer from nutritional deficiencies (due to anorexia, fad diets, or alcoholism) lack enough potassium. You need a daily minimum of 1,875 milligrams of potassium, and healthful extra virgin olive oil used in vegetable salads and stir-fries can help you get that. Take a peek at our Fruit Salad with Walnut Oil* and enjoy. Keep in mind, one cup of canned tomatoes contains 500 to 750 milligrams of potassium.

6 **Vitamin K:** Olive oil does contain a sufficient amount of this vitamin, which is important for bone formation because it binds calcium to the bone matrix. You need 70 to 140 micrograms of vitamin K each day. The best sources are spinach, parsley, and turnips. To get that dose of this bone-boosting vitamin, enjoy a spinach salad drizzled with olive oil.

OTHER OLIVE OIL INGREDIENTS

Aromatic substances: These are what give olive oil its taste and smell.

Coloring substances: These include carotenoids and chlorophyll, both of which have disease-fighting antioxidant benefits.

Hydrocarbons: These may be good for cholesterol, and their beta-carotene content has both vitamin A and antioxidant benefits.

Phytoestrogens: These may help beat bone loss as well as lessen hot flashes. In some Asian countries, where women consume plenty of phytoestrogen-rich soy, hot flashes are not common. (A bonus: Team soy with olive oil. I sailed though minor menopausal hot flashes by taking soy supplements.)

If you want to enhance your diet with photoestrogens, use olive oil, an edible phytoestrogen, with other foods that contain phytoestrogens, such as apples, asparagus, beans, blackberries, carrots, cherries, corn, flaxseed, garlic, green pepper, oat bran, onions, pears, squash, sunflower seeds, wheat germ, and yams. And yes, many of the heart-healthy recipes in this book include these foods.

Sterols: These may inhibit the absorption of dietary cholesterol.

Olive Oil Health Boosters

What It Is and Does	May Help Prevent
VITAMIN E: slows down the aging of skin and hair cells; helps to repair damaged muscle in the back; decreases free-radical damage.	Cancer (stomach, lung, larynx, esophagus), Parkinson's disease
VITAMIN K: reduces calcium and bone loss.	Osteoporosis
CALCIUM: maintains strong, healthy bones and teeth, which store 99 percent of the body's calcium; assists enzymes in fat and protein digestion and energy production; helps regulate the contraction of muscles, including the heart; aids the absorption of other nutrients.	Osteoporosis

Olive Oil Health Boosters (*cont.*)

What It Is and Does	May Help Prevent
IRON: plays a role in immune system functioning and is important to cognition.	Anemia
OMEGA-3s AND 6s: important for the lubrication of the joints; can serve as precursors for anti-inflammatory substances in the body such as prostaglandins (inflammation is one of the problems that contribute to asthma).	Heart disease, arthritis, inflammatory bowel disease, diabetes
POTASSIUM: plays a role in regulating blood pressure; balances out sodium levels to prevent water retention.	High blood pressure, heart disease, stroke, obesity

So, teaming olive oil with nutrient-rich foods is the way to go to enhance your total health. But how exactly does this liquid, once considered as good as gold, help your body to keep the doctor away and stave off disease? Scientists, medical doctors, nutritionists, and everyday people will show you how olive oil can be your best food friend—with no strings attached.

Honey, Citrus, and Olive Oil Fruit Kabobs

❖ ❖ ❖

GLAZE

½ cup honey
2 tablespoons lemon juice
2 tablespoons Cointreau
or any similar orange
liqueur

3 tablespoons extra virgin
olive oil
2 to 3 mint leaves, chopped

In a bowl, add the honey, lemon juice, and Cointreau; use a whisk to blend. Little by little, gradually whisk in the olive oil. Add mint and continue mixing. Reserve.

KABOB

8 bamboo sticks (6 to 8
inches)
8 cantaloupe or honeydew
wedges, cut in 1-inch
pieces
8 pineapple slices, cut in
1-inch squares

8 large strawberries
Powdered sugar for garnish
1 pint lemon fruit sorbet,
optional
Mint leaf

On each bamboo stick, place one piece of cantaloupe or honeydew, then a pineapple slice, and end with a strawberry. Arrange two kabobs on 4 serving plates; drizzle with the glaze. To serve, sprinkle kabobs with powdered sugar and decorate with a mint leaf. Serve with lemon fruit sorbet, if desired. Serves 4–8.

(*Source:* North American Olive Oil Association)

THE GOLDEN SECRETS TO REMEMBER

✓ Olive oil contains plenty of healthful nutrients.

✓ The quality of olive oil counts. Natural, organic, and made using the fast cold-pressed method is recommended by olive oil producers and medical doctors.

✓ Olives, from which olive oil is made, contain a variety of nutrients, including fiber, calcium, and vitamins A, C, and E.

✓ Essential fatty acids, the miracle workers of olive oil, help prevent heart disease and a variety of other diseases and health ailments.

✓ Olive oil contains antioxidants, calcium, iron, potassium, and vitamin K.

✓ Other good stuff, such as phytoestrogens and sterols, is also found in olive oil.

✓ The total ingredients of olive oil—especially when the oil is paired with a nutritious diet—can help prevent pesky health ailments and stave off life-threatening diseases.

Why Is Olive Oil
So Healthy?

*Olive oil is the best and safest of all oils. It
tastes good, too.*

—Andrew Weil, M.D.[1]

Once off the road, I put my wanderlust spirit to rest (like a
maturing olive tree in need of tender loving care and getting
a break from nature's harsh elements) and enjoyed serene
Mediterranean-like weather. But my curiosity of different
foods and different oils still intrigued me (as it did when I
was a kid in the suburbs).

In college, I was a nanny, of sorts, for affluent families in
the San Francisco Bay Area. One luxury home in Los Gatos
stands out in my mind. It was owned by a medical doctor and
his beautiful Italian wife, complete with three kids who lived
amid Mediterranean décor that I cherished.

In the kitchen, there was always fresh fruit and vegetables
somewhere in sight. In fact, the doctor's wife always sent me

home with a treat, whether it was guavas or lemons from their fruit trees in the front yard. And yes, there was the lingering aroma of garlic, and onions sizzling in olive oil in a large pan with a special dinner in the making.

I always felt a liveliness and feel-good vibe when I did my chores as I smelled the scent of good food throughout the house. And these days, I maintain that type of ambience in my own Tuscan-style kitchen (i.e., family-style wooden table, colorful Italian pottery, iron candle holders and hues of golds and reds) with something olive oil-based baking or cooking and fresh fruit and vegetables out on the countertops. It helps feed the body, mind, and spirit. What's more, there is proof that olive oil—the important food—is healthy.

Do you know that stacks and stacks of studies show that polyphenol-rich extra virgin olive oil can and does help to lower the risk of developing health ailments and diseases (at any age)? Here's a look at some research that you can put to work in your life to stay healthier.

8 HEALTH VIRTUES OF OLIVE OIL

1 **Cuts Risk of Heart Disease** For thousands of years, people around the Mediterranean Sea, including the residents of the Holy Land, have had lower rates of heart disease. The consensus is that olive oil is the common thread.

How Olive Oil Works: Studies show that a daily intake of olive oil lowers the risk of heart disease of all kinds, including heart attack. Olive oil has been shown to thin the blood, lower the blood pressure, and regulate cholesterol by reducing the "bad" kind (LDL) while maintaining the "good" kind (HDL). A healthful diet and lifestyle are key weapons in the battle to prevent heart disease—America's number-one killer for both men and women, according to the American Heart Association (AHA).

The good news is that olive oil may come to the rescue in America as it has for centuries in the Mediterranean world. Virgin olive oil may be more heart healthy than other vegetable fats, according to new research. European scientists have discovered virgin olive oil may help lower heart disease risk because of its high level of antioxidant plant compounds, according to a study published in the *Annals of Internal Medicine*.[2]

In a study of 200 young and middle-aged healthy men, three olive oils were used for three weeks. One oil was a virgin olive oil rich in poylphenols. The other two were processed with moderate to low polyphenols. The findings: The researchers discovered that polyphenol-rich virgin olive oil showed stronger heart-health effects than the more processed "nonvirgin" types. Virgin olive oil is more than just a heart-healthy monounsaturated fat. Polyphenols, claim the authors, may be the key to some of the health benefits linked to this healing oil. The scientific jury is still out, however, before the researchers recommend virgin olive oil as a replacement for other vegetable oils. And, not surprisingly, other health proponents favor using a variety of cooking oils.

What You Can Do: Both polyunsaturated fats (safflower, sesame seeds, soybeans, many nuts and seeds, and their oils) and monounsaturated fats (canola, olive, and peanut oils, and avocado) may help to lower your blood cholesterol and blood pressure when you use them in place of saturated fats in your diet, reports the AHA. (See Chapter 10, "The Elixir to Heart Health," for more studies and recommendations to lower your risk of heart attack and stroke, beat high blood pressure and cholesterol, and prevent or control diabetes.)

2 **Fights Cancer** While heart disease goes back to biblical times, cancer probably does, too. "Because of its aromatic oil content, olive oil is an effective antioxidant that has been shown to reduce cancer rates and increase longevity," points out *Healing Oils of the Bible*'s author, Dr. Stewart.[3]

In the twenty-first century, cancer is still a major threat for both women and men—and the threat of prostate cancer is a real one. Researchers at the University of California San Francisco discovered that men who ate more vegetable fat than less had a lower risk of dying from prostate cancer, which is a concern for men, even more as they age. Scientists studied nearly 4,600 men who had been diagnosed with prostate cancer back in 1986. After following these people for almost a decade, it was reported in *JAMA* that the men who ate more vegetable fat were less likely to die than those who did not eat it.[4]

How Olive Oil Works: Researchers at Copenhagen University Hospital in Denmark discovered that olive oil can reduce damage to cells, which can trigger cancer growth. For three weeks, 182 healthy men between the ages of 20 and 60 from five European countries consumed about one-fourth cup of olive oil every day. The findings: There was a 13 percent reduction in a marker of damage to cells. It's the phenols, believed to act as powerful disease-fighting antioxidants. In addition, the results (published in *The Federation of American Societies for Experimental Biology Journal*) may point to why the cancer rate is higher in northern Europe than in southern Europe, where olive oil is part of the olive-rich Mediterranean diet.[5]

Oleic acid, the main monounsaturated fatty acid in olive oil, as well as disease-fighting phenols may be the two primary components that lower the risk of developing skin, breast, and colon cancer.[6]

What You Can Do: The American Cancer Society (ACS) advises that you eat five to nine servings of fruits and vegetables daily to help lower your risk of developing cancer. Polyphenol-rich olive oil can help enhance the flavor of fresh produce, but the ACS does not validate olive oil used solo as a preventive measure for lowering the risk of developing cancer. But the ACS does note that lycopene, found in tomato products, does help in the prevention of some cancers, such as prostate cancer. Go ahead—enjoy vegetarian pizza or pasta with tomato sauce, because the effects of lycopene are increased when lycopene-rich vegetables are cooked and eaten together with fat.

3 **Wards Off Arthritis** Not only are there lower rates of cancer in the Mediterranean basin than in other countries, research in Greece also showed that the more fresh vegetables and olive oil people ate, the less likely they were to develop rheumatoid arthritis. Also, it's possible that the omega-3-rich fish eaten in a typical Greek diet may play a role in keeping stiffness, aches, and pains away, too.

Olive oil combined externally with soothing essential oils, which soothe muscle aches and pains, may have beneficial effects for arthritis aches and pains, often an age-related disease that can be worse in cold, damp climates. When I dined at Frantoio's, a staff member told me without hesitation that a regular customer vows that it's the extra virgin olive oil in his diet that keeps his arthritis at bay. I believed him.

How Olive Oil Works: Olive oil used daily may have anti-inflammatory benefits for pain by lubricating joints and reducing swelling. Also, folk doctors believe eating cooked antioxidant-rich vegetables with olive oil provides polyunsaturated and mono-unsaturated fats that are used by your body to make the good prostaglandins that reduce swelling and pain.

What You Can Do: Include olive oil in your daily diet. While some folks use olive oil on their salads and cooked vegetables and eat fish to help stave off arthritis, others turn to olive oil paired with essential oils in massages to loosen up stiff muscles and joints.

4 **Keeps Diabetes at Bay** Diabetes (type 2), like arthritis, has been a problem for a long time. Worse, the numbers are soaring for both baby boomers and senior citizens. We can blame high blood sugar on a high-fat diet, excess weight, and a sedentary lifestyle.

How Olive Oil Works: It's believed that olive oil can cut the amount of "bad" LDL cholesterol as well as triglycerides, also known as fats, in your blood. This, in turn, may help to lower your risk of developing type 2 diabetes, which can be controlled by making diet and lifestyle changes. Olive oil may also lower your blood sugar. Why? The good effect may be due to olive oil being a monounsaturated fat. And there's more.

Consuming three tablespoons of extra virgin olive oil each day can cut your odds of developing diabetes, recent Spanish researchers suggest. Adults at risk for heart disease who eat a Mediterranean diet rich in olive oil can lower their risk of developing diabetes. In a study published in *Annals of Internal Medicine*, more than 3,500 men and women between 50 and 80 benefited from EVOO. It may be due to the anti-inflammatory effect and antioxidants.[7]

What You Can Do: Eat a low-fat, heart-healthy "fishatarian" diet, which is plant-based, low in fat, and full of whole grains, legumes, fruits, and vegetables. Keep your weight in check, and do not overdo your intake of olive oil, since a high-fat diet can lead to weight gain and other health problems.

5 **Stops Pain** Diabetes is often painless, especially before it gets out of control, but pain can be a pain in the rear. "Olive oil has also been used as a healing ointment for centuries by Greeks, Romans, Egyptians, Christians, and Jews. While usually combined with essential oils, it was routinely applied to cuts, sores, bleeding wounds, bruises, and injuries of all kinds, with a little wine as antiseptic," notes Dr. Stewart.[8]

How Olive Oil Works: Research shows that olive oil contains a chemical, oleocanthal, that can stop inflammation similar to painkillers such as ibuprofen and other anti-inflammatory medications.

What You Can Do: Use olive oil topically to help heal cuts, sores, and other ailments that involve inflammation, redness, and pain. Also, it couldn't hurt to include olive oil in your daily diet as well, since it may help to strengthen your immune system and speed up the healing process. Plus, we know that omega-3s can help reduce inflammation, which often creates pain.

6 Inhibits Loss of Memory While none of us wants to be in physical pain, mental illness can be a nightmare, too. Alzheimer's is a brain disease that affects brain function. Its symptoms include tearjerker film–like loss of independence and relationship woes, as depicted in *On Golden Pond* and *The Notebook,* in which characters are trapped in their bodies as their minds and memories deteriorate.

How Olive Oil Works: Researchers at Columbia University Medical Center in New York studied about 2,000 adults (in their mid-seventies) including 194 who had Alzheimer's disease. They studied what the people ate in the year prior to the onset of the disease. The findings were that the closer a person's eating habits were to the Mediterranean diet, the lower his or her odds were of having Alzheimer's. The diet may help reduce brain inflammation and oxidation in the body. The monounsaturated acids are believed to maintain cell structure and membranes in the brain.[9]

That's not all. More research shows olive oil can protect the brain.

A bit of olive oil and nuts may help protect the brain. Studies continue to tout incorporating a Mediterranean diet into your life. It may help keep your mind clear, a path to brain wellness, scientists in Spain reported in the *Journal of Neurology, Neurosurgery & Psychiatry*. Kudos may be due to the heart-healthy diet with monounsaturated healthy fats, which may lower odds of damaging inflammation, fight plaques found clogging the brains of people with Alzheimer's disease, and improve brain blood flow. These brain health benefits—including better cognitive skills—were found in 7,400 people at high risk of heart disease because of diabetes.[10]

What You Can Do: Include olive oil, an important monounsaturated fat source, in a Mediterranean-type diet.

7 **Beats Bone Loss** Losing your mind can be a challenge, but bone loss can be debilitating as well. The connection between bone density and fracture was made back in the late eighteenth century by Ashley Cooper, who coined the term "osteoporosis," once considered an old woman's problem. But nobody is immune.

How Olive Oil Works: The main polyphenol in olive oil, oleuropein, may prevent bone loss with inflammation. Olive oil is also believed to assist calcium absorption and to help beat bone loss and even reverse the crippling effects of osteoporosis. If your diet is deficient in calcium, your body will steal it from your bones. This will weaken your skeleton and can lead to the brittle bone disease. Fats such as olive oil are needed for proper calcium metabolism and are essential components of cartilage and bone, say nutritionists.

What You Can Do: While calcium is needed to fight osteoporosis, olive oil (which has a small amount of this mineral) can help supplement your intake of it when teamed with calcium-rich, bone-building foods.

8 Defends Against HIV In the early 1980s, HIV hit the world and caused a panic more than all of the above diseases combined ever did. The question "What if it becomes a widespread epidemic?" haunted people around the world—of both genders. If you have human immunodeficiency virus (HIV), it can lead to acquired immune deficiency syndrome (AIDS), which can be spread to other people through the exchange of body fluids through sex, blood transfusions, and sharing of needles. There still is no cure.

How Olive Oil Works: While HIV—the cause of AIDS—has led to countless deaths globally, a new buzz is circulating. A compound called maslinic acid (a natural product derived from olive-pomace oil) may help to slow down the spread of HIV.

Researchers at the University of Granada believe that olive-pomace oil can slow down the spread of AIDS in the body by 80 percent. The product inhibits serine protease (an enzyme used by HIV to spread the infection throughout the body).

What You Can Do: Include olive oil in a well-balanced, nutrient-rich diet to keep your immune system in working order and fight off infections.

Take-10 Super Cookies

❖ ❖ ❖

Super, because they're moist, chewy, and packed with tasty ingredients. "Take-10" because 10 of those ingredients* (marked with an asterisk) are considered by cancer researchers to be "breast-cancer friendly." Including them in your diet is a good start toward preventing breast cancer. In the end, these cookies aren't to die for . . . they're to LIVE for.

*⅓ cup (2⅜ ounces) canola oil

1 cup (7½ ounces) brown sugar

½ teaspoon baking powder

¼ teaspoon baking soda

*1½ teaspoons ground cinnamon

*1 teaspoon ground ginger

*¼ teaspoon ground cloves

¾ teaspoon salt

2 teaspoons vanilla extract

1 large egg

2 tablespoons (1½ ounces) boiled cider (for great flavor; substitute maple syrup or dark corn syrup, if desired)

*1 cup (3½ ounces) shredded fresh carrots

*½ cup (3 ounces) semisweet or bittersweet chocolate chips

*½ cup (2 ounces) dried cranberries, packed

*½ cup (2 ounces) blanched slivered almonds, toasted in a 350° oven till golden, 9 to 12 minutes

*1 cup (4¼ ounces) King Arthur White Whole Wheat Flour, organic preferred

*1½ cups (4¾ ounces) quick rolled oats

Preheat your oven to 350°. Lightly grease (or line with parchment paper) two baking sheets.

In a large mixing bowl, combine the oil, brown sugar, baking powder, baking soda, spices, salt, vanilla extract, and egg, beating until smooth. Add the boiled cider or syrup. Stir in the carrots, chocolate chips, cranberries, and almonds, then the flour, beating gently until well combined. Add the oats last, making sure they're thoroughly distributed throughout the bowl.

Drop tablespoon-sized balls of dough onto the prepared sheets, leaving about 1½ inches between them. Bake the cookies until they're just barely set on top—about 12 minutes. Remove them from the oven and cool them on the baking sheets; they'll be very soft, so don't try to transfer them to a rack. Once cool, store in a covered container, with waxed paper or parchment paper between the layers to keep the cookies from sticking to one another. Yield: About 30 cookies.

(*Source:* King Arthur Flour)

In the next chapter, I'll show you how the Mediterranean diet and its components, such as olive oil, come into play for good health—and why following this diet and lifestyle for life can be a good change to make today for tomorrow for you, your children, and their children to follow. It truly seems to be a key to good health. (Also, in Chapter 12, "Antiaging Wonder Food," I'll explain how some of these diseases can be controlled with olive oil and other preventive measures.)

THE GOLDEN SECRETS TO REMEMBER

OLIVE OIL KEEPS THE DOCTOR AWAY

Disease	How Olive Oil Works
√ Heart disease	Polyphenols in extra virgin olive oil help to lower the risk of heart disease of all kinds.
√ Cancer	Phenols in extra virgin olive oil act as disease-fighting antioxidants to hinder the cancer process; oleic acid may reduce the growth of tumors.
√ Arthritis	Omega-3s in extra virgin olive oil may play a role in reducing aches and pains because they may have an anti-inflammatory effect.
√ Diabetes	Olive oil may cut the amount of "bad" LDL cholesterol as well as triglycerides in the blood, which may lower the risk of developing type 2 diabetes.
√ Pain	Oleocanthal in olive oil can stop inflammation similar to the way painkillers do.
√ Impaired memory	Monounsaturated acids maintain cell structure and membranes in the brain.

OLIVE OIL KEEPS THE DOCTOR AWAY (*cont.*)

Disease	How Olive Oil Works
√ Osteoporosis	Olive oil helps calcium absorption, which is needed to beat bone loss.
√ HIV	Maslinic acid (a natural product derived from olive-pomace oil) may help to slow down HIV.

The Keys to the Mediterranean Diet

Cleopatra and Nefertiti knew the wonderful effects of olive oil. Natural cosmetics are in. The Mediterranean lifestyle is in, and, thanks to cooking shows on television, olive oil is in. It's that simple.

—Margot Hellmiss[1]

I was on a new journey, in my mid-twenties, commuting to San Francisco State University (trying to be productive like an olive tree in a grove) and settling down to study and live a domesticated life with a male companion, a foodie, who had Italian descendants and had introduced me to the wide world of good European eats—olive oil, Italian bread, cheeses, nuts, vegetables, spices, and herbs. I had left counting calories on the road.

This boyfriend of mine was a full-blooded Italian. One of the traits he possessed was that he loved to cook good, hearty

Mediterranean food. I was living on a shoestring in a down-town Victorian studio in San Jose, California. It was charming but sparse. After all, I was a starving student. But when he prepared dinners, I always felt like royalty.

One night in particular, my personal chef began the process of making a spaghetti sauce to die for. The ingredients, fresh tomatoes, garlic, onions, and olive oil, remind me of the noteworthy prison dinner scene in the film *Goodfellas*. In other words, it doesn't matter where you live but it matters how you put together a meal that sizzles. The heart and soul of the Mediterranean diet and lifestyle, whether you are from Italy or Greece, make cooking and eating a decadent pleasure.

I bet you think I'm going to discuss the popular Mediterranean diet books. Not me. I've discovered in my research that for thousands of years, olive oil—and other key factors—have played a major role on the Greek island of Crete, where Cretes and other Greeks live longer than other people in the world.

In fact, according to the World Health Organization, in 2004, the life span of men and women in Greece ranked second, with Italy third. Japan was number one, and the United States trailed behind.[2]

It turns out that the way I've been eating for decades (that is, fresh fruits, vegetables, potatoes, nuts, seeds, bread and other cereals, and yogurt) is nothing new. However, using more "good" olive oil and more saturated fat is new to me, since I'm a boomer of the 1950s, when meat and potatoes were a constant on the average dinner table and butter was replaced by margarine.

The fascinating thing is, while olive oil is a fat (120 calories per tablespoon), and other foods in the Mediterranean diet are high in fat, heart disease is lower and the longevity rate higher in European countries such as Greece and Italy than in America, where our fat intake is often lower. This is called the "French paradox," and it continues to work for people who follow the traditional Mediterranean diet. But for those who stick to the American diet and eat "bad" fats, unwanted body fat is the end result.

FIGHT FAT WITH FAT

When I was in my early forties, I discovered that while I looked skinny, I was fat. I recall that at this time, I was working out at the gym on a regular basis. While I was eating plenty of vegetables, fruits, and whole grains, I skipped the fish and "good" fats. A bodybuilder, Anna, noticed that my muscle mass wasn't in tip-top shape. Plus, the gym's nutritionist measured my body fat—not good.

So, I tweaked my diet big-time. I dumped the non-fat foods and blue cheese salad dressing into the trash. I began to eat nuts, tuna, salmon, and eggs, and I drizzled vinegar and olive oil on my salads and sandwiches. As I continued my new, improved Mediterranean-type diet and lifestyle, teamed with faster long-distance walking and more serious weight lifting, within weeks I noticed a difference in my muscle definition. Not only did I lose 5 pounds, but I built muscle and had a new, improved body, with sculpted arms and legs as well as normal blood pressure. I give credit to losing the "bad" fats and welcoming fish, eggs, fat, and a new exercise routine—all part of the Mediterranean diet.

10 KEYS TO THE MEDITERRANEAN DIET

These dietary tips, straight from Oldways Preservation & Exchange Trust, will help you to get on the right track to following a healthful, heart-healthy Mediterranean diet without feeling like you're on a diet.

TIP 1: Eat plenty of food from plant sources, including fruits and vegetables, potatoes, breads and grains, beans, nuts, and seeds.

TIP 2: Focus on a variety of minimally processed and, wherever possible, seasonally fresh and locally grown foods to get health-boosting and disease-fighting anti-oxidants.

TIP 3: Use olive oil as a primary fat, replacing other fats and oils (including butter and margarine). Surprise: In Chapter 8, "More Healing Oils," discover the health perks of butter (in moderation.)

TIP 4: Aim for a daily total fat amount ranging from about 25 to 35 percent of energy, with saturated fat composing no more than 7 to 8 percent of calories.

TIP 5: Consume low to moderate amounts of cheese and yogurt (low-fat and non-fat versions are best).

TIP 6: Eat low to moderate amounts of fish and poultry, and zero to four eggs per week (including those used in cooking and baking).

TIP 7: Enjoy fresh fruit as your daily dessert, and limit sweets with a sugar (often honey) or saturated fat to no more than a few times per week.

TIP 8: Consume red meat a few times per month. Lean cuts are preferable.

TIP 9: Get regular exercise, which will help you maintain a healthy weight, fitness, and well-being.

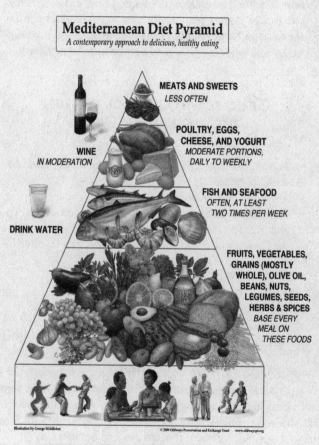

Mediterranean Diet Pyramid
A contemporary approach to delicious, healthy eating

MEATS AND SWEETS
LESS OFTEN

**POULTRY, EGGS,
CHEESE, AND YOGURT**
*MODERATE PORTIONS,
DAILY TO WEEKLY*

WINE
IN MODERATION

FISH AND SEAFOOD
*OFTEN, AT LEAST
TWO TIMES PER WEEK*

DRINK WATER

**FRUITS, VEGETABLES,
GRAINS (MOSTLY
WHOLE), OLIVE OIL,
BEANS, NUTS,
LEGUMES, SEEDS,
HERBS & SPICES**
*BASE EVERY
MEAL ON
THESE FOODS*

Illustration by George Middleton   © 2009 Oldways Preservation and Exchange Trust   www.oldwayspt.org

BE PHYSICALLY ACTIVE; ENJOY MEALS WITH OTHERS

TIP 10: If you drink alcohol, opt for moderate consumption of wine, normally with meals. Limit intake to about one to two glasses per day for men and one glass per day for women. Note: Alcohol should be avoided during pregnancy and whenever it would put the individual at risk.

GOOD-FOR-YOU FOODS OF THE MEDITERRANEAN DIET

- *Bread, pasta, grains:* Bread, pasta, rice, couscous, polenta, potatoes
- *Fruits:* Olives, avocados, grapes
- *Vegetables:* Spinach, eggplant, tomatoes, broccoli, peppers, mushrooms, garlic, capers, beans, legumes, nuts, pine nuts, almonds, chickpeas, white beans, lentils, olive oil
- *Cheese and yogurt*
- *Fish:* Shellfish, sardines
- *Poultry:* Chicken
- *Eggs*
- *Sweets:* Pastries, ice cream, cookies
- *Meat:* Veal, lamb

In addition, daily physical activity is recommended. Getting physical can include doing chores, group activities, solo activities, fun stuff, and gym workouts. In other words, everyday lifestyle activities teamed with exercise is good for you head to toe, according to researchers and doctors.

Olive Oil on the Side

There are easy ways to fit an hour's worth of exercise (up to 500 calories burned) throughout your day by dividing it up into 10- or 15-minute segments. Just rev up your energy when doing everyday housework or chores—and don't forget the olive oil.

Chores	Calories Burned per 30 minutes	Olive Oil
Sitting (watching TV)	30	Read *The Healing Powers of Olive Oil, Revised and Updated,* and learn new ways to maintain your weight by eating fat and fat-burning foods
Sleeping	30	Put olive oil on your feet
Washing the dog	97	Use a tablespoon of olive oil before shampooing

Chores	Calories Burned per 30 minutes	Olive Oil
Raking leaves	98	Use olive oil on the rake to prevent rust
Painting the house	136	Use olive oil to remove paint from your skin
Chopping wood	150	Use olive oil–based soap afterward
Mowing the lawn	178	Use olive oil on the mower to prevent rust
Gardening	180	Spray indoor plants with olive oil and water
Scrubbing the floor	188	Use a solution of water and olive oil to clean the floor
Shoveling snow	195	Eat a pasta dish with olive oil for energy

According to the American Heart Association, "there's no one 'Mediterranean' diet. At least 16 countries border the Mediterranean Sea. Diets vary between these countries and also between regions within a county." However, the people of these various Mediterranean countries share these dietary components: high consumption of fruits, vegetables, bread and other cereals, potatoes, beans, nuts, and seeds; olive oil as an important monounsaturated fat source; dairy products, fish, and poultry consumed in low to moderate amounts and little red meat eaten; eggs consumed zero to four times a week; and wine consumed in low to moderate amounts.[3]

While the Mediterranean-style diets are similar to what the AHA recommends, they are not identical. In other words, the diets of the Mediterranean region do contain a high percentage of calories from fat. This is believed to be the cause of an increase of obesity in these countries.

The AHA points out that both heart disease and life span in the Mediterranean countries are lower than in the United States. They also note that "but this may not entirely be due to the diet. Lifestyle factors (such as more physical activity and extended social support systems) may also play a part." Before the AHA advises people to turn to the Mediterranean diet, more research is needed.

The Mediterranean diet isn't called heart healthy for no reason. Study after study, including another one published in *The New England Journal of Medicine*, show that the diet that continues to get top diet rankings in the United States by different reports, staves off heart attacks and strokes. About 30 percent of deaths from these two top killers may be prevented if people switched to the longevity-boosting Mediterranean diet—and olive oil plays an integral role since it is the recommended primary fat with myriad healing compounds.[4]

A bowl of pasta with vegetables and drizzled with olive oil may be the perfect remedy to aging gracefully for middle-aged women, like me, and perhaps you, too, now or one day. Researchers studied the diet and health of more than 10,000 women in their late 50s and early 60s. Checking back 15 years later, those women who followed the Mediterranean diet, like I preach and follow, were healthier as they aged. So here is more proof that enjoying vegetables, whole grains, and, of course, olive oil—and tossing out processed foods and eating less meat—can be the prescription to living a longer, healthier life for women.[5]

While I believe olive oil plays a big role in good health, I have also shown you that it's just part of the health package—it is not the only reason Europeans have lower rates of heart disease than Americans. Also, olive oil is ranked high as a superior healing oil, but take a look at Part 3, "Other Natural Oils," to see how olive oil's cousins—flavored oils (herbal, spice, vegetable, citrus, and other fruits) and other types of healing oils—can help you in other remarkable ways, too.

Panzanella
(Bread Salad with Vegetables)

❖ ❖ ❖

Bread salad is a very good way to use up Italian or French bread that has gotten too hard. To make homemade bread crumbs, use a food processor or blender.

½ pound Italian bread, several days old
⅓ cup lemon juice or wine vinegar
Oregano to taste
½ cup Marsala Olive Oil
1 teaspoon Dijon mustard
6 green onions (white part) chopped
4 garlic cloves (or to taste) minced
Salt, pepper, and paprika to taste
½ cup fresh basil or parsley, chopped
6 tomatoes, chopped (red or yellow)
2 tablespoons capers
2 bell peppers, roasted, diced
1 cucumber, sliced thin
1 cup green beans or asparagus, cooked crisp tender
1 or 2 avocados sliced (for top)
1 cup olives (for top)
1 cup cherry tomatoes (for top)

Soak bread in cold water about 5 minutes. Squeeze to remove excess water. Place in large, shallow serving bowl. In the jar of the blender, whirl together vinegar or lemon juice, oregano, olive oil, mustard, green onions, garlic, paprika, salt, pepper, and basil. Add tomatoes, capers, bell peppers, cucumber, and beans to the bread in a bowl. Pour oil mixture over ingredients; toss gently. Arrange avocados, olives, and cherry tomatoes on top to garnish. Serves 6 to 8.

(*Source: Cooking with California Olive Oil: Treasured Family Recipes* by Gemma Sanita Sciabica)

THE GOLDEN SECRETS TO REMEMBER

✓ Research shows that a low-fat diet does not lower health risks.

✓ The "French paradox," or eating a diet richer in fat combined with antioxidant-rich fruits and vegetables, may help lower your risk of developing cancer and heart disease.

✓ Research shows there is no reason to deprive yourself of "good" fatty foods such as fish and olive oil.

✓ The Mediterranean diet—food from plant sources—can help stave off heart disease.

✓ The Mediterranean diet includes using olive oil as a primary fat.

✓ Regular exercise and moderate consumption of wine (if you drink) are also included in the traditional healthy Mediterranean diet.

PART 3

OTHER NATURAL OILS

Flavored Olive Oils

*The strands of spaghetti were vital, almost alive in
my mouth, and the olive oil was singing with flavor.*
—Lucien Tendret[1]

One Thanksgiving, my boyfriend with Italian roots and I
were invited to his mother's home in Santa Cruz, a popular
beach town (in a coastal region where south-central California olive trees flourish), for a dinner. Instead of a snowy
November day with classic holiday dishes, such as turkey and
pumpkin pie (the traditional dishes I was familiar with from
childhood), I was introduced to fog and gray skies at dusk.
The elegant table fit for royalty in a European country had
me at first sight. The zillion course meal was served in the
dining room (bigger than our apartment) with an earthy table
setting complete with the scent of vanilla candles and red and
white roses set off with a panoramic view of the Pacific
Ocean—the cold water I had bodysurfed in during the sixties.

The dishes, from appetizer, sides, entrée, and dessert, included crostini, Mediterranean fruit salad, duck, French bread
dipped in olive oil, chocolate cheesecake, and espresso. Each
food boasted herbal notes and citrus flavors—lemon, lime,

orange, and tangerine. It was a delectable feast to move me—
and it did.

I finally asked her the question (much like I did with
Florence, the Italian lady who had baked me cookies with her
treasured olive oil): "The meal is delicious. What's your secret?" I was curious to know why each dish was a masterpiece.
"Flavored olive oils," she told me. And, to this day, I recall and
cherish the ambience and the foods enhanced with olive oils.

Combine fresh herbs and spices with olive oil and what do
you get? Healthful flavored or infused olive oils can offer an
extra punch to your health and taste buds. Just ask Jonathan
Sciabica, a member of the Sciabica family, which is well-
known in the olive oil world for their products. He had this to
say about their jalapeño olive oil: "This innovative combination of fresh jalapeños and Mission olives is a break from any
conventional olive oil. Nick Jr. enjoys using this olive oil to
fry his eggs in the morning. This won't really burn your tongue
like a jalapeño might but you'll get a kick, and the flavor of
the pepper comes through in the most amazing way."

Like healing olive oil, popular herbs and spices—such as
jalapeño, oregano, and rosemary—boast health benefits, too.
You can make your own flavored oils and reap a variety of
therapeutic rewards from these herbs and spices mixed with
extra virgin olive oil. Plus, it's most likely a rewarding experience to make your own flavored concoctions—sort of like
growing your own vegetable garden.

Interestingly, "Olive oil which has had herbs or fruits infused in it cannot be called olive oil. According to International Olive Oil Council regulations it must be called 'fruit
juice.' In reality, few producers comply with this and you will
see labels such as 'lemon infused olive oil' or 'basil olive oil.'
Because of their immense popularity, the California Olive
Oil Council is trying to come up with a meaningful labeling
standard for flavored oils," explains John Deane, M.D.

Meanwhile, I took Gemma Sciabica's advice and combined herbal, spice, and fruit "olive oils" in one chapter. At first, I was going to discuss herbal oils and fruit-flavored oils in separate chapters. So, read on—and discover some of the delicious concoctions you can add to your diet.

HEALING HERBAL AND SPICE OILS

Here, take a look at some of the favorite and cutting-edge herbs and spices that are infused in olive oil, as well as some information and news about their healing powers.

CHICORY (*Cichorium intybus*): The Eygptians and Greeks drank roasted chicory root to relieve stomach, liver, and kidney complaints. A tonic made from chicory root is believed to increase the flow of bile, which is good for staying regular.

GARLIC (*Allium sativum*): It's an ancient healing food. During biblical times, garlic was praised for its versatile uses, including as a diuretic, a sedative, an anti-inflammatory, and a cure for internal parasites, and in poultices.

JAPALEÑO (*Capsicum annuum*): It's capsaicin, the hot stuff, that may help slow down cancer cell growth, clear sinus congestion, soothe a migraine, act as an anti-inflammatory, and make aches and pains go away. Hot peppers also have antioxidants A, C, and E.

OREGANO (*Oregano vulgare*): Oregano oil is both antiseptic and anti-inflammatory. Not only does it kill bacteria, viruses, fungi, and other germs, but it also fights infection, from colds to the flu.

PARSLEY (*Petroselinum crispum*): Parsley can be traced back to Greek mythology. Legend has it that it was a bad omen for a soldier to see it before going to battle. But things have changed. This cleansing herb is packed with disease-fighting antioxidant vitamins A, C, and E. Also, it boasts plenty of iron. Parsley gets its good reputation, however, for its diuretic action. Plus, it's believed to ease PMS symptoms, including cramps, hormonal mood swings, and bloating.

ROSEMARY (*Rosmarinus officinalis*): Rosemary is believed to cure headaches, hemorrhoids, depression, and other ailments that take a toll on your total health and well-being. This ancient therapeutic herb contains calcium, magnesium, sodium, and potassium, all of which help balance fluids surrounding the nerves and heart tissues. In fact, rosemary may help to lower blood pressure. The rosemary leaf may also have other positive health effects.

SAGE (*Salvia officinalis*): This camphor-flavored "fountain of youth" grows wild in the Mediterranean. Its Latin name means "to heal or save." Legend has it that sage will add years to a person's life if used regularly. Herbalists claim sage is a natural astringent and antiseptic. It's recommended for gingivitis and sore throats. Note, however, that women should not take it.

THYME (*Thymus vulgaris*): Thyme is a delicate herb that is a natural source of iron, magnesium, silicon, sodium, and thiamine. Its power is as an antiseptic and a general healing tonic. It can also subdue coughing and relieve intestinal ailments.

Make Your Own Flavored Olive Oils

You can purchase ready-made infused olive oils or make your own flavored oils by blending your favorite herbs and spices. The safest way is to use dried herbs. Sure, you can use fresh ingredients (and actually, I would prefer to do just that), but caution is advised. Why? Simply put, it's risky business to put anything in the oil that contains water. That means, be on alert when teaming olive oil with garlic, lemon peel, fresh peppers, fresh herbs, or spices. The fact is, the oil won't support bacterial growth, but the water-containing herbs will. Worse, botulism bacteria can grow in this type of environment. (Yes, botulism can make you very ill.) But note, there are several ways to have your homemade flavored oils and survive, too. Here, take a glance at four tips that can help you do it yourself:

- Mix all the ingredients. Then, put the prepared oil in the fridge and use it within one week. Go ahead—add whole cloves of garlic, lemon peel, fresh or dried peppers, ginger, rosemary sprigs, or whatever strikes your fancy.
- Preserve the added ingredients. Maybe you have seen garlic or herbs mixed with olive oil. The way it is done commercially is to first preserve the water-containing garlic or herb in a strong brine or vinegar solution, then put it in the olive oil. The vinegar solutions used commercially are up to four times stronger than the vinegars you find in the supermarket. You can

find them at commercial food supply outlets. Many of the herb mixes have both salt and vinegar, both of which prevent bacterial growth.

- Dry the herbs to remove all the water, leaving the essential oils. This can be done using a food dehydrator or just by leaving them in the sun. Then, add the spices and herbs to the olive oil.

- Press the olives with the spices. Putting lemon, garlic, and other ingredients in the olive press with the olives is the safest way to flavor olive oil. *Note:* The glitch is that you have to have your own olive press or go to a commercial press. The oils from the added ingredients mix with the olive oil, and the watery parts of the spices are removed along with the olive water. You can mix a small amount of oil with the fresh ingredients, let the flavors mingle, and then decant the oil, leaving the herbs and any water behind. Mix this flavored oil with a larger amount of oil. You can also add essential spice oils to the olive oil to achieve the same effect.

Caution: It is difficult to determine the exact shelf life of homemade flavored olive oils. American Dietetic Association (ADA) nutritionists question their safety, since we do not know if we can prevent food-borne illnesses. So caution is advised.

HEALING CITRUS OILS

Citrus olive oils—lemon, lime, orange, and tangerine—are new and exciting to me. Personally, I have already tried a commercial brand of lemon olive oil. One night, I tossed some in a pasta dish. While it wasn't homemade, it did add zest to my pasta plate. Still, there is a wide world of citrus olive oils . . .

I do know that lemon—a fresh, light, and cool scent—was used in ancient times to perfume clothes and repel insects. Europeans used lemons to fight infectious illnesses such as malaria, and English sailors turned to lemons as a scurvy remedy. You can use lemon for its light and zingy benefits. If you're feeling down and blue, it can pick up your spirits. This oil is used in beauty products, soaps, and household cleansers.

One man in particular really knows his flavored oils, and it shows in his book *Michael Chiarello's Flavored Oils and Vinegars* (Chronicle Books, 2006). He writes, "Some lemon oils made in Tuscany are extraordinary. Whole lemons are ground along with the olives into a paste and then pressed, extracting the lemon flavor with the oil. In this process, the lemon and olive flavors become joined in a way impossible to duplicate in the home kitchen. These oils also tend to be fabulously expensive. Home-made oils emphasize the fresh, juicy character of citrus and are a particular delight for summer cooking."[2]

Here, take a look at an easy-to-do lemon olive oil recipe that spells "fresh" from the get-go.

Lemon Olive Oil

❖ ❖ ❖

1 lemon
2 cups Marsala Olive Fruit Oil

Peel lemon with vegetable peeler. Place peel and olive oil in glass container and cover. Bring to room temperature before serving. Keep refrigerated for several days.

(*Source: Cooking with California Olive Oil: Treasured Family Recipes* by Gemma Sanita Sciabica)

Chiarello explains in his book that the flavors of citrus oils "are essentially interchangeable." I suppose that is true unless you happen to love lemon and lime as I do. But in a pinch, the flavored olive oil is all right. "If I run out of orange," he says, "I just fill out the amount in the recipe with lemon. When using citrus oil, you are adding the flavor but not the acid."[3]

I'm not surprised that Chiarello adds that citrus oils are superb when paired with salads—and you don't need vinegar. Also, he adds that citrus-flavored olive oils are different from the concentrated citrus essence oils on the market and that you can't use them in the same ways, such as in baking, to flavor cakes and cookies. (I use lemon olive oil to grease dishes when baking scones and brownies.)

Spiced Citrus Whitefish Tacos

❖ ❖ ❖

*½ pound white fish fillets
    (such as halibut or
    mahimahi), skinless
2 tablespoons lime olive oil
2 tablespoons jalapeño
    olive oil*

*4 tablespoons orange juice,
    divided
¼ teaspoon sea salt
¼ teaspoon black pepper*

FOR TACOS

*4 corn tortillas
Shredded purple cabbage
Thinly sliced onion*

*Chopped fresh cilantro
Sour cream
Grated orange zest*

Preheat grill or broiler. Place fish in a shallow baking dish. Whisk together oils, 2 tablespoons orange juice, salt, and pepper; pour over fish and turn to coat. Let sit at room temperature, 20 minutes, turning once. Place fish directly on grill on under broiler. Cook until fish flakes easily, about 8 minutes, turning once. Let cool 5 minutes; flake fish, toss with remaining 2 tablespoons orange juice and set aside.

Assemble the tacos: place a corn tortilla on each serving plate. Top with cabbage, onion, cilantro, and flaked fish. Top with sour cream and orange zest. Serve immediately. Serves 4.

(*Source:* The Olive Press)

Now that we've put some favorite flavored oils on the table (in Chapter 18, "The Joy of Cooking with Olive Oil," discover which foods go best with flavored olive oils), let's talk about other healing oils that are used inside and outside the body.

THE GOLDEN SECRETS TO REMEMBER

✓ Chicory   Relieves stomach, liver, kidney ailments

✓ Garlic   An anti-inflammatory, a diuretic, a sedative

✓ Jalapeño   Slows cancer growth, clears sinuses, soothes aches

✓ Oregano   Antiseptic and anti-inflammatory, relieves muscle soreness

✓ Parsley   Cleanser, diuretic

✓ Rosemary   Heart-healthy, cancer-fighting

✓ Sage   Astringent, antiseptic, soothes sore throats

✓ Thyme   Antiseptic, helps anemia, suppresses coughs, relieves stomach upsets

More Healing Oils

*We know consumers recognize the various types
of dietary fats but have a hard time determining
what types to increase or decrease in their diet.
This provides an opportunity to encourage consumers to choose foods rich in healthful fats
such as plant-based oils.*

—Susan T. Borra[1]

Nontraditional Thanksgiving dinners, like the one I savored
and shared with you in the last chapter, made me more ap-
preciative of sophisticated food. I began to feel big-time
guilt with drive-through fast-food fixes. One windy fall afternoon in San Francisco, I cut my Nutrition 101 class and
took a detour to the student union. I drank diet sodas for the
caffeine effect and analyzed why I dodged taking the test on
fats and oils. I didn't get it. On the floor, sitting cross-legged
in jeans and a SFSU sweatshirt, I watched the soap operas
All My Children and *One Life to Live* and wrote a story for

my favorite creative writing class. But the topic of dietary oil was on my brain.

Each time I peeked at the big book on foods, I flipped the pages to the section on oils and fats—and I got lost. It was complicated. The "un"-fats left me confused like math. I tried to comprehend what fats were good and what fats were bad. It was easier to close the book and go order french fries. Ironically, in retrospect, I was devouring soda with zero fat and consuming trans fat fries. Still, I was clueless to my eating habits gone bad. I flunked the nutrition class (blame my failure on oil), but I managed to maintain a mandatory 3.0 plus in my major of English (creative writing).

Years later, when I wrote the first edition of *The Healing Powers of Olive Oil*, I took a refresher class of sorts from Gemma Sciabica, the olive oil producer's wife and cookbook author of five books, in central California. During our dangling conversations (dominated with food and how to prepare it), the octogenarian became my mentor and taught me, phone call after phone call, that you can cook and bake anything with olive oil.

Gemma has baked cookies for me. One time for a book signing, I didn't feel confident making cookies using olive oil, and they arrived on my doorstep in the nick of time. It's true. The Sicilian fig cookies were moist and my favorite. I'll never forget the day the box arrived, and I had wanted these cookies in particular. It took me back to my dear friend Florence, who had baked me biscotti. Gemma could have made any kind, from hundreds of her recipes, but she sent these fig gems. I screamed out of excitement, and these treats didn't leave the house—they were for me and me only.

Recently, one afternoon in the fall, I confessed to her again (as though she were a priest; we are both Catholic) that I combine butter—all kinds—with olive oil in my dishes. She told me back in the twentieth century, she (a home chef ahead of her time) did use olive oil as did chefs in Europe and the United States who created Mediterranean dishes. Also, to my surprise, Gemma admitted that she does use a small amount of butter to spread on toast and agrees with me that the flavor is rich. While olive oil continues to get attention for its health benefits, other essential oils (and even butter) are in the limelight, too. Still, Gemma is a proponent of olive oil and her health and longevity prove that the oil deserves to be number one in healing oils.

In my college days—the first time around, in junior college—I recall taking a nutrition class. I was fascinated with calories and staying fit (it was in the 1970s, and staying clear of fat and looking skinny like fashion models in *Cosmopolitan* and *Vogue* magazines was "in"). But, I flunked the lesson on fats. I remember it was confusing—fats such as saturated, polyunsaturated, and monounsaturated. At the time, to me, it was boring. It was a foreign language.

TALKING "GOOD" FATS IS IN STYLE

These days, people around the world are talking about "good" fat. Not only is olive oil hot stuff, but other oils are now also the talk of the town. Why? Food chains from Starbucks to Kentucky Fried Chicken (KFC) are jumping on the "good"-fats bandwagon and deleting trans fats—and choosing other types of oils for their fried and baked foods.

KFC, for one, is turning to a new soybean oil—a neutral-tasting, all-purpose, organic oil. Soybean oil contains both omega-3 and omega-6 fats as well as good-for-you monounsaturated fat and saturated fat. To reach zero trans fat, Starbucks is replacing butter with a trans-fat-free margarine and a butter–trans-fat-free margarine blend. "There is, however, the possibility that certain items may have trans-fat-free vegetable oils (such as soy or canola oil) but this is not broadly used in our fresh baked products," said company spokesperson Alan Hilowitz.

So, now that popular food chains are getting fat-savvy, read on to get a handle on some of the cooking oils. (See Chapter 11, "The Olive Oil Diet," to learn more about how unhealthy trans fats can not only be harmful for heart health, but can pack on the pounds, too.)

ALL FATS ARE NOT CREATED EQUAL

Type of Fat	Oils	Effects on Your Body
Saturated	Coconut oil, palm kernel oil	Raises both LDL and HDL cholesterol
Polyunsaturated	Vegetable oils: corn, sesame, soybean	Reduces both HDL and LDL cholesterol; too much may raise cancer risk
Monounsaturated	Canola oil, olive oil, peanut oil	Lowers LDL, HDL stays the same or may be raised depending upon the individual
Trans fatty acid	Margarines, vegetable shortenings	Raises LDL, lowers HDL

SUPER OILS, SUPER HEALING, AND COMMON COOKING OILS

At first when I tackled this topic, I thought, "I will create a list, Top Healthiest Oils, and rank them from 10 to one." But after pondering a group of oils, I decided no way. Each cooking oil I dish about boasts health perks. Also, "good" fats may change to "bad" in the land of nutritional gurus and controversy as time passes. So if I rave about coconut oil and announce it's my number-one favorite oil, the odds are one day one scientist may create a one lab-rat study on the pros and cons of the exotic oil. The findings: It may be a sequel of the film *Charley*. The rat will expire, and my oil kudos will be under scrutiny like a lab rat.

To be balanced when it comes to discussing cooking oils, here is a working list of good working oils that are likely here to stay for a variety of health benefits. But note, new, improved cooking oils—or old ones—could create a shake-up in the world of oils that goes back to the beginning of time.

Also, I left out corn oil (my mother used Mazola as an all-purpose oil, from cooking to deep frying in the seventies) and cotton oil. These two oils have some health perks, but they are full of omega-6 fatty acids, which may trigger inflammatory diseases if you overindulge. So I decided to pass as I would, too, if cooking or baking with either of the shaky oils.

Welcome to my world of tried-and-true cooking oils (I've used them in cooking, baking, and topically, too) that I enjoy. But I also look forward to experiencing other oils used around the globe.

Lorenzo's Oil (Olive and Rapeseed Oil)

Remember the 1992 film *Lorenzo's Oil*? The story is about an uncommon debilitating disorder called adrenoleukodystrophy (ALD), which, in nearly half of cases, destroys the nerves in the brain. Young boys who are affected, such as Lorenzo Odone, usually become disabled (it can look like multiple sclerosis) and often die sooner than later.

One remedy is Lorenzo's oil, which is made from olive and rapeseed oils, teamed with a low-fat diet. While the oil has not been proven to be a wonder drug, Lorenzo Odone celebrated his twenty-eighth birthday in 2006. According to the www.washingtonpost.com, on January 28, 2007, Lorenzo was still alive at 28. He died May 30, 2008.

Interestingly, rapeseed oil, a monounsaturated fat, is high in both omega-3 and omega-6 fats. Still, the "healing" oil has a bad reputation because some people claim the oil may cause health problems, due to its component of erucic acid. Some people are also concerned about canola oil, which has a very low level of erucic acid.

Almond Oil

Oil Roots: Almond oil goes way back to the beginning of time of the almond nut. Its oil was used by the Greeks and Romans for massage. Not to forget: The almond tree is a gift of the nut, and is enjoyed for its wide array of medicinal virtues.

Healing Powers: Not everyone knows almond oil boasts monounsaturated fats. Olive oil and other nut oils get a lot of attention, so it seems this oil is often put on the back burner except with masseuses. The thing is, though, almonds rich in omega-3s and protein are super healthy, and there are stacks of studies to prove this fact.

Best Uses: Years ago I discovered the wide world of essential oils. Almond oil, a base oil, is used for massage recipes. While it's touted for its topical use, it's also used in the kitchen as a versatile cooking oil.

Taste Tests: Like other healing oils, such as olive oil, it's rich in monounsaturated fats, which play a big role in the Mediterranean diet, an underlying theme in my *Healing Powers* series. I use many nut oils in cooking and baking, but I have yet to use this oil in my dishes.

Avocado Oil

Oil Roots: Avocado oil, like almond oil, is another of my personal favorites. It is a versatile oil, as well as an edible one, pressed from the fruit of the avocado. Not only is it used in food but it also is found in products like moisturizing lubricants and cosmetics.

Healing Powers: Rich in monounsaturated fats, it can help the body absorb lycopene and beta-carotene—the good-for-you antioxidants. It may also boost good cholesterol.

Best Uses: Health gurus, from M.D.s to R.D.s, claim salads, sandwiches, and dips are healthy paired with avocado, so it's safe to say avocado oil could be good, too. But because it is high in fat, moderation is key to maintain an ideal weight.

Taste Tests: A container of avocado oil is in my pantry. My first experience with it was on a tossed green salad. Instead of olive oil, I used the avocado oil in a homemade salsa and guacamole. While avocado slices aren't my favorite food, they are doable and nutritious with fresh greens—especially Mexican food. Using the oil is a good way of getting its goodness and bypassing the slippery texture that reminds me of sci-fi snake films.

Canola Oil

Oil Roots: While avocado oil is new to me, canola oil goes way back in time. Canola oil is believed to be derived from both rapeseed and brassica oilseed—which has a history of being used for oil lamps centuries ago, as well as in Asian countries. In the twenty-first century, canola oil can be found in the grocery store aisles as an oil blend, combined with sunflower and soybean oils. And it is also infused in butter and a variety of food products.

Healing Powers: Recent research shows canola oil fights belly fat. American and Canadian researchers discovered oleic vegetable oils like canola oil may lessen girth around the middle, as well as lessen the risk of developing metabolic syndrome (a cluster of health problems including high blood sugar, blood pressure, and cholesterol) that can trigger heart disease, stroke, and type 2 diabetes. Credit goes to monounsaturated fats. A study of 121 people at risk for metabolic disorder drank a smoothie full of one and a half ounces of one of five oils, part of a 2,000 calorie per day diet. The findings presented at the American Heart Association's 2013 Scientific Session in New Orleans showed the people who used canola oil (not the corn/safflower combo) for one month enjoyed a change of 1.6 percent less belly fat. More research is needed, but while the jury is out, a bit of canola oil in your diet regimen along with regular exercise is healing oil for thought.[2]

Some people confuse canola oil with rapeseed oil (which contains erucic acid that can be unhealthy). But canola is derived from the canola plant—which also contains erucic acid but is approved by FDA standards.

Taste Tests: Several years ago at the tail end of the twenty-first century, I used canola oil as versatile all-purpose cooking oil, from greasing a pan for an omelet to baking bread with it. Also, before I wrote *The Healing Powers of Olive Oil* (first edition), I was taken by soft margarine containing canola oil. I used it as a spread for toast and bagels, in pasta, and on French bread. It tasted good, or so I told myself because of the heart-healthy factor, and I ignored liquid fats, such as extra virgin olive oil and other healing cooking oils. And I shunned my favorite friend—real butter—which I missed dearly.

Coconut Oil

Oil Roots: Canola oil is an all-purpose oil that most people have heard of if not used, but coconut oil is a cooking oil that is getting new attention and for good reason. This ancient tropical cooking oil is growing in popularity in the twenty-first century—not just on exotic islands, either. It, of course, is derived from the meat of coconuts harvested from the coconut palm.

Best Uses: It is available in liquid and capsule form. Virgin coconut oil keeps its scent and taste of coconut. The shelf life is up to two years.

Taste Tests: Where have you been all my life, coconut oil? I first used coconut oil by including it in baked goods, from pies to cookies. Later, I graduated to stir-fries and appreciated the tropical oil for its monounsaturated fats, superb flavor, and its multiple uses for eating as well as body care.

Two Timeless Oils

Evening Primrose Oil

Oil Roots: The evening primrose (*Oenothera biennis*)—a plant with bright yellow flowers—is found in dry meadows from the Atlantic to the Rocky Mountains. It blooms only in the evening—hence the name "evening primrose"—then dies, leaving seed pods, which can be used for their oil.

Healing Powers: Evening primrose oil contains gamma-linolenic acid (GLA), an essential fatty acid. Some medical experts believe GLA is the most important essential oil for treating PMS and menopausal symptoms.

Research suggests that women with PMS or menopausal woes have low levels of GLA. It's been theorized that such a deficiency might cause a prostaglandin deficiency and trigger a sensitivity to prolactin, the pituitary hormone. GLA supplementation may relieve the prostaglandin deficiency.

Not only is prolactin involved in the menstrual cycle and the ending of it, so are the hormones progesterone and estrogen, which can affect water retention, breast swelling, irritability, and breast tenderness. The GLA from evening primrose oil may help to balance these fluctuating hormone levels.

Best Uses: Many women take evening primrose oil capsules fourteen days before their period to relieve PMS symptoms. Evening primrose oil is found in health food stores.

Fish Oil

Oil Roots: Eskimos in Alaska and Greenland eat cold water fatty fish as a staple in their diet. This has resulted in their having fewer problems with cancer and heart disease, which affect people who use unhealthy fats.

Healing Powers: Fish oil is rich in the omega-3 fatty acids EPA and DHA. Fish oil can be helpful for arthritis because the omega-3 oils are important in the lubrication of the joints. They also reduce pro-inflammatory chemicals called prostaglandins. Some holistic doctors believe that a diet high in the essential fatty acids is brain food. EFAs can help the cell membranes work in the brain.

The omega-3s are diabetes fighters because they can help control the blood sugar and help prevent damage to all tissues. Also, the omega-3s are essential fatty acids that have protective effects on heart disease. And, not surprisingly, Dr. Barry Sears' *Omega Rx Zone: The Miracle of the New High Dose Fish Oil* (Regan Books, 2002) touts fish oil for better health.

Best Uses: Fish oil capsules are taken as a supplement and are helpful for people who do not get an adequate amount of the omega-3 fatty acids EPA and DHA. But note, do not take high doses of fish capsules if you are taking NSAIDs (nonsteroidal anti-inflammatory drugs). They may increase gastrointestinal ulcers and bleeding.

Flaxseed Oil

Oil Roots: Flaxseed was discovered as a food by the Greeks and the Romans. This plant with turquoise blue blossoms is hailed because of the oil that comes from its seeds and the many health virtues that oil provides.

Coconut oil won me over, but healthful flaxseed oil (a woman's best friend) still has yet to make it into my diet regimen. But it has a lot of health perks, according to research—I should rethink adding it to my oil repertoire.

Healing Powers: Flaxseed oil is Mother Nature's best source of alpha-linolenic acid, an omega-3 essential fatty acid—the same healthful fatty acid in fish oil that boosts heart health, reduces inflammation, and enhances cell function in your body. Medical experts also believe it can be a woman's best friend. Why? It has been known to aid in PMS and menopausal woes. It also lowers cholesterol and blood pressure, and may help lower the risk of developing heart attack and stroke.[3]

Best Uses: Flavorful flax oil can be a healthful replacement for butter. But note, it is not good for cooking because high heat will destroy the good-for-you nutrients of the oil. Go ahead and use this oil as a flavoring for potatoes, vegetables, and popcorn. Also, nutritionists recommend adding flax oil to smoothies, yogurt, and salad dressing.

Taste Tests: I've been a smoothie fan for decades. So it made sense to healthy it up with a bit of flaxseed oil. While pesky, out-of-sync hormones are in my past, it's worth using the heart-healthy oil that may fight the winter blues, too. I put a teaspoon in a blackberry smoothie complete with organic milk, all-natural ice cream, and berries. No, I didn't taste anything different, but I felt I got a nutritional boost.

Grapeseed Oil

Oil Roots: Health nuts are familiar with flaxseed oil and most likely know of another multiuse healing oil, too. Welcome to grapeseed, also known as grape seed, oil, which is pressed from the seeds of grapes, and it's no surprise it's not uncommon with winemakers.

Grapeseed oil (also called grape oil) has been used for thousands of years by people in European countries. These days, grapeseed is produced in Italy, France, and Spain. Its versatile appeal has made it a common oil for cooking and baking, to make flavored oils, and massage oils, and in hair products, lip balm, hand creams, and sunburn repair lotions.

Healing Powers: Unlike olive oil, grapeseed oil, high in heart-healthy monounsaturated fat, is mainly polyunsaturated and not recommend for cooking. But it is good served cold on foods and in baked goods. Speaking of good, grapeseed oil is believed to increase good HDL cholesterol and lower bad LDL cholesterol, thanks to its antioxidants.

Best Uses: Grapeseed oil can be used for sautéing, medium-high-heat frying, and baking [and oil infusing (i.e. flavored oils)]. Grapeseed oil is excellent for cooking, since it can be brought to a higher heat and has a milder taste than extra virgin olive oil. This cooking oil is best for using as a base for salad dressing; it's commonly infused with herbs, such as garlic and rosemary as well as spices, too. Health-conscious folks are familiar with this oil, but it's yet to make a splash in mainstream America.

Taste Tests: I got this cooking oil at our local health food store. Making homemade waffles and pancakes is easy, and the flavor is better than the frozen kind. It seemed like the right thing to do to add a bit of grapeseed oil to my pumpkin waffles—and I did just that.

Hempseed Oil

Oil Roots: Getting acquainted with grapeseed oil is one thing, but meeting hempseed oil (no, it's not marijuana, so you will not get a buzz) is another oil experience that is well worth the discovery. The hemp plant has grown in many regions for thousands of years. While its descendants are from the same plant as marijuana, it's not the drug. You can get health benefits from both hempseed oil and hempseeds, much like flaxseed oil and its seeds.

Healing Powers: Omega-3 and omega-6 acids are essential fats the body can't make, and it's up to you to find foods, like hemp oil, which are good sources and have balanced ratios of omega-6 and omega-3 to stay heart healthy. Also, it's believed the ideal ratio may help in both artery healing and as anti-inflammatories—gamma-linoleic acid (GLA) and omega-3 fats—which may help lower your risk of stroke. Hemp oil, like hempseeds, may also lower triglycerides and cholesterol levels (the stuff that can cause heart attacks) as well as help keep your blood pressure numbers in check.

Best Uses: It's healthiest to use this oil on salads and vegetables. You can find it online or at health food stores. Note to self: Mix in cooked cruciferous vegetables and brown rice. (I will not heat it due to some folks claiming this oil is best not used in baking or cooking.)

Taste Tests: In my kitchen cabinet this oil, like flaxseed oil, is one that I can benefit from but am hesitant to try. It's an acquired taste like 70 percent cacao chocolate. I haven't tried it as of yet (it sits next to my favorite healing oils, including avocado and macadamia nut oil), but that doesn't mean I won't open the can. Its health perks are truly too good to ignore.

Macadamia Nut Oil

Oil Roots: Adding flaxseed oil and grapeseed oil to my pantry made me feel like I was expanding my healing oil repertoire. But macadamia nut oil is just a fun and good-for-you oil that I loved including in my diet—and doesn't require an acquired taste. Another favorite healing oil of mine, macadamia nut oil is expressed from the nut meat of the macadamia tree found in Australia.

Healing Powers: The fact is, olive oil is not the only oil that is monounsaturated plentiful—so is macadamia nut oil, and it even boasts more! Like olive oil, this nut oil is part of the heart-healthy Mediterranean diet. Omega-3 fatty acids lower triglyceride levels and raise HDL "good" cholesterol numbers.

Best Uses: This healing nut oil is versatile in the kitchen for healthful salads as well as sautéing, and used for beauty care, too. It can be used in many dishes, whether you bake or cook with it. By consuming it, however, you're going to keep your heart healthy.

Taste Tests: My first experience with macadamia nut oil was as an anti-frizz beauty hair care product. The inexpensive oil is shocking. One day when I was hit by dry hair in the winter, I put a small amount in the palm of my hand and onto my long, curly locks, and immediately the dryness was AWOL. I also have baked muffins and breads and added this popular nut oil. It has a nice aroma, and the taste is not over-powering. It's a breath of fresh oil in my pantry.

Peanut Oil

Oil Roots: While I've used sweet macadamia nut oil, peanut oil is one oil I've witnessed in films where characters use it in recipes (to kill off characters with nut allergies), including cake. Peanut oil, also known as groundnut oil, is derived from pressed peanut kernels. It has Spanish roots but is used in Asian cuisine, such as Chinese and South Asian foods. The oil can be refined, unrefined, cold-pressed, but it's the roasted kind that bears a strong peanut flavor.

Healing Powers: Antioxidant E is sometimes added to peanut oil because of its preservative merit. Like almond oil, it is used as a massage oil. Due to its monounsaturated fat, it can lower bad cholesterol and increase good cholesterol. What's more, peanut oil contains resveratrol, the heart-healthy compound found in both wine and red wine vinegar.

Best Uses: The most common usage of peanut oil is in stir-fried seafood and vegetables and very healthy, steamed vegetables. It could prove good also in chop suey, moo goo gai pan, and steamed dumplings.

Taste Tests: When I envision peanut oil, I believe it would prove flavorful in a peanut butter cookie of a nutty, sweet type of recipe, as well as in a vegetarian's stir-fry. Because it lends to a versatile nature, it will find a place in my pantry. It can be ordered online and found in Asian specialty shops.

Pumpkin Seed Oil

Oil Roots: Peanut oil is not to be passed up (I will use it for its cooking appeal), and as a devout pumpkin lover, pumpkin seed oil is one that will be used by me sooner than later with no doubts. It is made by pressing roasted, hulled pumpkin seeds from pumpkins. It has been appreciated in Austria since the 1700s.

Healing Powers: Folk remedy followers believe it battles inflammation due to its omega-3 fatty acids and vitamin E (an antioxidant), like other healing oils. There are no double-blind groundbreaking research studies that say it can help lessen the pain of arthritis, but people will tell you aches and pains may be less than more, thanks to the decrease in swelling.

Best Uses: Since this healing oil contains good-for-you nutrients, it makes sense that it is useful in the kitchen. Pumpkin seed oil can be used in salad dressings and is especially nice for colder seasons like fall and winter. That way, you will not compromise its antioxidant value. But why not use it in pumpkin dishes, like pie and cake and casseroles?

Taste Tests: Since I love pumpkin pie and pumpkin-spiced coffee, of course pumpkin oil is in my pantry. I found it at my local health food store, but it's also available online. I used it in a late autumn stir-fry to get that warm, light-colored "green-gold" nut flavor mixed in, with flavorful fall vegetables, like zucchini, tomatoes, and whole grain pasta.

Red Palm Oil

Oil Roots: Unlike nut and seed oils, exotic red palm oil is less popular in the United States. It's an edible vegetable oil and palm oil that comes from the fruit of oil palms, found in Africa, southeast Asia, and Brazil. Its cooking benefits go back in time; its health perks are beginning to collect a following around the world.

Healing Powers: Healthful red palm oil is not the hydrogenated palm oil found in processed foods. True red palm oil is high in saturated fat, but it is also high in monounsaturated fat, like both good-for-you macadamia nut oil and olive oil. Red palm oil boasts vitamins A and E. It also contains plenty of beta-carotene—and that's why its color is reddish orange.

Best Uses: Naturally, you'll want to add it to your diet, but this gets tricky. Red palm oil proponents recommend not cooking with it because of loss of antioxidants. That means drizzle it on cooked foods, like vegetables and soups.

Taste Tests: I was looking forward to trying this vegetable oil. Once I opened the jar, I was surprised that the oil is semisolid—like coconut oil. My mission was to drizzle it on a whole-grain-flavored organic popcorn. I tasted the carroty flavored oil and turned to melted honey and grass-fed cow butter. My use of red palm oil will most likely be mixed in with cruciferous vegetables or a homemade vegetable soup.

Rice Bran Oil

Oil Roots: Pumpkin seed oil had me at *pumpkin,* but rice bran oil has made its way into my vegetarian-based diet, too. Let me introduce you to rice bran oil, aka rice extract, which is the oil extracted from the germ of the inner husk of rice. It's a popular cooking oil in Asian countries, such as China and Japan.

Healing Powers: This healing oil truly boasts some healing powers. It contains a hodge-podge of antioxidants, including vitamin E and phytosterols. It's believed that consuming the oil may improve cholesterol by lowering bad LDL and raising good HDL cholesterol levels. Some folks who believe in folk medicine claim it may help lessen hot flashes during menopause. But I'm thinking it could be because it's teamed with a healthful diet.

Best Uses: Since rice bran oil boasts a high smoke point, it is a good oil with a mild flavor, perfect to use in vegetable stir-frying with fresh herbs to add more disease-fighting antioxidants. And vegetables contain estrogen, which may also help with being a natural remedy to stave off pesky hot flashes.

Taste Tests: I have a large plastic container of rice bran oil in my kitchen cupboard. More times than not, I have cruciferous vegetables, onions, and garlic ready to use for all occasions. When I used rice bran oil for the first time, I didn't notice the taste. I did include herbs, spices, and a bit of butter. So I got my taste buds satisfied and added good-for-you oil.

Safflower Oil

Oil Roots: Rice bran oil works for me, but safflower oil—not so much at this time, but that doesn't mean it should be ignored. A more popular cooking oil than rice bran oil is safflower oil. It's derived from the safflower plant, which is cultivated for vegetable oil. It's extracted from the seeds and goes way back to the beginning of time. This plant grows in India, Mexico, the United States, and dozens of other countries.

Healing Powers: This oil is a great source of monounsaturated oleic fatty acid. Actually, there are two types of oils: the monounsaturated type is used for hot dishes. The polyunsaturated is best on nutrient-dense fresh salads with seasonal vegetables.

Best Uses: The monounsaturated type of safflower oil is recommended for hot dishes because of its high smoke point. The polyunsaturated kind is best drizzled on cold salads, completed homemade sauces, and cooked vegetables. Since it has a lack of distinct flavor, this cooking oil is best married with other flavorful oils.

Taste Tests: Back in the twentieth century, I recall seeing this type of cooking oil kept in our kitchen cupboard. I didn't reach for it then (lard and margarine were my choices), and with all these other healing oils, I still haven't used it.

Sesame Seed Oil

Oil Roots: Like peanut oil, sesame seed oil is linked to southeast Asian cuisine. It comes from sesame seeds. Interestingly, this oil goes back in time before 600 BC when Sumerians and Assyrians used it for massages, food, and medicinal salve.

Healing Powers: Sesame seed oil boasts both monounsaturated and polyunsaturated fat contents, which can be added to a heart-healthy diet. This healing oil is rich in antioxidants.

Best Uses: Sesame oil has a place in Asian cuisine. It's finding its way to the United States and mainstream grocery store shelves. It is best added to dressings, marinades, and like peanut oil, it fares well in stir-fries.

Taste Tests: Its medium smoke point makes sesame seed oil a good healing oil candidate for sauces and baking—which attracts me, and I can see using it in a sweet bread, home-made bagels, rolls, and sweet and savory muffins.

Soybean Oil

Oil Roots: So I passed on safflower oil, but as one who has nibbled on soybean nuts, this vegetable oil extracted from the seeds of the soybean may make its way into my life. It is one of the most widely consumed cooking oils, most likely for its versatile use, price, and adaptability.

Healing Powers: Vegetable oils, like this one, are made with soybeans, and that in itself makes it a go-to oil for both monounsaturated and polyunsaturated fats.

Best Uses: Soybean oil has not too low and not too high of a smoke point—it has a nice medium cooking ability, which makes it a fine choice for healthful vegetable sauces and stir-fry dishes. Better still, there is no overpowering aroma or taste, so while you get its health perks, you won't have to hold your nose to do so.

Taste Tests: I haven't tried this oil, but soybean nuts have made their way into my diet as have vegetable stir-fry recipes. Since it is veggie-friendly, I will make it a point to add it to my healing oils stash.

Walnut Oil

Oil Roots: Soybean oil will be in my kitchen cupboard and stir-fries, but walnut oil already has made it into my homemade baked breads. It is extracted from English walnuts. It's basically found and produced in France and my Golden State, California.

Healing Powers: These versatile nuts boast heart-healthy omega-3s, which are also good for brain wellness as well as being mood boosters. That means walnut oil, also rich in protein and vitamin E, can help you chase away winter blues and summer sadness and deal with the ups and downs in life.

Best Uses: It's believed walnut oil is good used in salads and cooked vegetables, and as a nut oil, I can agree. I can personally attest that I've used walnut oil in baking, whether it be with breads or muffins.

Taste Tests: The oil doesn't have an overpowering flavor, so it doesn't change aroma or taste in foods, such as vegetables and fish. The bottom line: I do use it in a variety of ways and pray I may get a little bit of help from its promise of super mood-enhancing and brain-boosting powers.

There are numerous cooking oils that I did not mention.

COOKING OILS AT A GLANCE

Medical doctors, nutritionists, and chefs will tell you that olive oil is not the only healing oil, since the following oils have great benefits, too. To find out more about cooking and baking with these healing oils, refer to Chapter 19.

Oil	What It Does
Almond oil	A good carrier oil for essential oils used for massage
Avocado oil	An up-and-coming heart-healthy oil high in monounsaturated fat and good cholesterol
Canola oil	A popular oil, like olive oil, that is rich in monounsaturated fat. It contains heart-healthy omega-3s.
Coconut oil	An immune enhancer; an oil that is healthful for your outer body beauty, from hair to skin, because of its rich moisturizing benefits
Flaxseed oil	A high-lignan oil that relieves depression, fatigue, and allergies. Lignans are estrogen-like substances that have balancing effects on serotonin and other mood regulators.
Grapeseed oil	An antioxidant-rich oil that might help prevent diseases, such as cancer and high cholesterol
Hempseed oil	Heart-healthy with GLA and omega-3 fats
Macadamia nut oil	Rich in heart-healthy monounsaturated fats.
Peanut oil	A protein source rich in vitamin E to help stall aging
Pumpkin seed oil	This oil is high in health-promoting essential fatty acids, magnesim, and protein.
Red palm oil	High in vitamin E and beta carotene
Rice bran oil	This disease-fighting antioxidant rich oil is becoming more popular in the twenty-first century.
Safflower oil	An all-purpose cooking oil, but its

	omega-6s need to be balanced with omega-3s for heart health.
Sesame seed oil	Good for drizzling on antioxidant-rich vegetable stir-fry dishes
Soybean oil	Another oil boasting monounsaturated fat and polyunsaturated fats—good for heart health
Walnut oil	A nut oil with a variety of healing powers, from boosting heart health to boosting brain wellness

Note: Check with your doctor before using any of these oils in case there's a medical reason they're not right for you.

Speaking of healing oils, in Part 4, "Youth in a Bottle," you'll learn how teaming vinegars (especially apple cider vinegar and red wine vinegar) with olive oil is another Mediterranean secret to losing body fat, maintaining your weight, and stalling age-related diseases such as heart disease.

SPECIALTY OILS IN THE LIMELIGHT

Other cooking oils, including argan oil and black truffle, are attracting attention, especially with chefs. Argon oil is a deep golden-colored oil. It's lighter in weight than nut oils and olive oils. Like sesame oil and pumpkin oil, it is used in Morocco. It can be a special treat for salads, fish, and vegetables. It is used also for both hair and skin benefits, as well as in cleansing and antiaging products. It can be found in specialty shops and online.

Like argan, black truffle oil is unique and gaining merit. Often, this rich cooking oil is infused with black truffles (a fruiting body of a fungus) or olive oil. It is best used drizzled over food. It is recommended to use on french fries, in pasta dishes, or on mashed potatoes. It is popular because truffles can be pricey, so this makes black truffle oil a delicacy. It contains the same health perks as olive oil. It is used in Middle Eastern, French, Spanish, Italian, and Greek cuisine.

Butter: The New "Health Food"

Pass the butter, please! Several years ago, after I penned the first edition of *The Healing Powers of Olive Oil*, I confess I bought butter. I ate it on the sly. I could have written a real-life book on *Confessions of a Butter Eater*.

One day I told my dear friend/olive oil producer's wife Gemma Sciabica, "I like to bake with it."

She darted, "It's animal fat."

And, of course, being a health author and devoted health nut, I listened to the woman decades my senior, and sensed she was right, sort of. After all, olive oil has a record of being heart healthy and can add years to your life. But I continued to buy, eat, and cook/bake with rich European-style butter. Ironically, both my blood pressure and weight maintain the same numbers. So I have pondered, "Is real butter, like dark chocolate and coffee, good for you used in moderation?"

Desperately seeking to be thin, too many of us have gone fat-free "crazy," but haven't shed the unwanted pounds. Worse, some people have gained weight on no-fat diets. The reason is that fat-free foods contain sugar and calories, but we gobble them up thinking that they're okay because they're fat free. I recall years ago, I'd buy "healthy" margarine with less calories. Not only did it taste like cardboard, I rebelled and became a closet butter eater.

How much butter should you eat? It's a no-brainer you're not going to stay lean and heart healthy if you eat a stick of butter daily. But note, if you don't eat enough fat, such as butter, you'll end up unsatisfied and eventually you'll go off your diet plan. That's why you should incorporate a small amount of fat, such as butter, into your daily diet. Past research compared a low-fat diet with a high-fat diet (mostly from good fats). After time, high-fat eaters lost pounds, and low-fat dieters gained pounds. The reason, according to researchers: Fatty foods, such as avocado, chocolate, nuts, olive oil, and butter curb hunger by satisfying the desire for some fat.

But I didn't need a study to give me permission to eat butter. For several years to present-day, I incorporated flavorful butters with olive oils while sautéing vegetables and baking muffins. Not only did my dishes taste better by pairing the oil and fat, but I was hardly alone. I noticed chefs in the Mediterranean countries back in the twentieth century combined butter and olive oil, too.

Enter my world of butter, a by-product of milk. That means it's 80 percent fat, and the rest is water and milk solids. Butter is a mix of fats: saturated, monounsaturated, and polyunsaturated. It boasts some calcium, potassium, and plenty of vitamin A.

The World of Butter: Good butter can help make great sauces, cakes, pastry, candy, and cookies. Butter can be salted or sweet, and chefs favor unsalted butter for its mild flavor. Speaking of taste, European-style "cultured" butters are what I favor and use in my recipes. True, they are higher in fat, but for taste's sake, they're worth it.

Then there is ghee, clarified butter, which has had the water and milk solids removed so it is 100 percent fat. It has a longer shelf life and higher smoke point than regular butter—it is welcomed in the Paleolithic diet, the stuff hunters and gatherers ate centuries ago during the cavemen era. Its foods include fish, lean meat (not in my vocabulary), fruits and vegetables, and staying clear of dairy, grains, legumes, sugar (these are my favorite foods), and salt. Olive oil, coconut oil, and honey are part of the thumbs-up caveman-era foods, too—and this type of eating style is gaining attraction in the twenty-first century.

Lastly, it is important to add that butter from grass-fed, organically raised cows is the healthiest butter you can eat. And yes, I have it in my fridge. It's an acquired taste. (I use it to sauté vegetables and spread on whole grain toast and bagels.) Butter with roots in grass-fed animals contains CLA (conjugated linolenic acid), a healthy fat believed to help lower your risk of developing cancers—and it may even help you keep belly fat at bay.

Research Backs Butter: Thanks to the saturated fat in butter, a study published in the *British Medical Journal* suggests that butter—and cheese—may be not all that bad. London researchers argue that trans fats in fast foods, bakery products, and margarines up heart disease via the inflammatory process. (In November 2013, the FDA discussed banning the use of trans fats. Food items flaunt "no trans fats" on packaging, so there is growing consumer awareness of its unhealthy nature.) People believe Ancel Keys' study "demonized" saturated fat, and its usage plummeted. The findings were that saturated fats have little weight on your risk for developing heart disease and stroke. Evidently, the scientists claim past research hasn't supported a link between saturated fat and heart disease. Instead, saturated fat has been found to be protective. What's more, turning to a Mediterranean diet after a heart attack is almost three times as potent in reducing mortality as taking prescription medication.[4]

Please note, I use butter, cheese, and other saturated fat foods (both in the past twentieth and twenty-first century) but indulge in moderation, *and* like good chefs, pair them with healing oils to get the variety of taste and health benefits. (Go back and reread Chapter 3, "A Historical Testimony" and Chapter 6, "The Keys to the Mediterranean Diet.") So, yes, I'm out of the closet. I believe butter is a "good fat," just like olive oil, coconut oil, avocado oil, and other healing oils in this chapter are good foods. The bottom line: Butter is a health food if you treat it with respect, like eating the right kind of chocolate—and less is more. Yes, you can have your butter and eat it, too!

California Healthy Granola Bars

❖ ❖ ❖

Flashback to 1999 during the Y2K hoopla. I befriended dozens of granola bars in boxes (the hippie health snack in the sixties) just in case the world ended as we knew it. My pantry was stuffed with these survival goods infused with good-for-you superfoods. My neighbors visited me to look at my stockpile and laughed at me. Once 2000 rolled in around the globe and the scare was over, the countless uniform bars (peanut butter and chocolate chip) were devoured by me, one by one, day by day, as I dealt with winter woes and craved instant energy. Store-bought bars, like these, were doable but lacked flavor. These multi-oil-infused granola bars, my own recipe, are chewy, a bit crumbly, and semisweet, complete with healing oils for a twenty-first-century twist.

1¼ cups quick-cooking rolled oats
½ cup light brown sugar
¼ cup honey
1 organic brown egg, beaten
½ cup pancake and baking mix
2 tablespoons organic 2-percent low-fat milk
1 tablespoon each flaxseed oil, coconut oil, and butter

1 cup mix of dried apricots, cranberries, and plums
½ cup dark chocolate chips
¼ cup sunflower seeds
1 capful pure vanilla extract
½ teaspoon ground cinnamon
½ teaspoon allspice
1 tablespoon orange- or lemon-flavored olive oil
Shredded coconut (topping)

In a bowl, mix oats, brown sugar, honey, egg and baking mix. Add milk, oils, and butter. Fold in fruit, chocolate chips, seeds, vanilla extract, and spices. Pour mixture into an 8-by-8 square baking dish lightly greased with flavored olive oil. In a 350° oven, bake for about 20 minutes or until golden brown and firm. Cool. Sprinkle with coconut. Slice into rectangle bars. Serves 12. Place in plastic container with lid, preferably in the refrigerator or freezer.

THE GOLDEN SECRETS TO REMEMBER

✓ Saturated oils—such as coconut oil and palm kernel oil—aren't heart healthy, so be sure to use them in moderation.

✓ Polyunsaturated oils—vegetable oils such as corn and

sesame—reduce "bad" cholesterol, but using too much can up your risk for developing cancer.

✓ Monounsaturated oils—canola oil and olive oil—are the healthiest fats.

✓ Trans fatty acids—margarines and vegetable shortenings—are unhealthy, artery-clogging fats that can cause heart disease and weight gain.

✓ Canola oil contains heart-healthy omega-3s and is a good fat choice.

✓ Evening primrose oil and flaxseed oil are good oils for women because they can help in coping with hormonal woes such as PMS and menopausal symptoms.

✓ Fish oil—rich in both omega-3s and omega-6s—can help prevent heart disease, diabetes, and other health problems.

✓ Grapeseed oil, high in disease-fighting antioxidants, can stave off heart disease and cancer.

✓ There is a wide variety of cooking oils that include fruits, nuts, and soy.

✓ Some nut oils, such as almond oil and walnut oil, are heart healthy.

PART 4

YOUTH IN
A BOTTLE

Combining Olive Oil and Vinegar

If you pour oil and vinegar into the same vessel,
you would call them not friends but opponents.
                                    —Aeschylus[1]

As a college student (like a growing olive tree in a farmer's grove showing promise), I savored cheese and chocolate with their feel-good ingredients and fat (good and bad) and avoided olive oil. But that doesn't mean olive oil didn't make its way into my diet when I was a teenager introduced to a school of new foods. On a hot and sunny Sunday afternoon complete with a bright blue sky, typical for the Silicon Valley, my family was invited to dinner at my godparents' home, which was also in the suburbs but across town in an upper-middle-class neighborhood. And this was when I met face-to-face no-nonsense foodies who introduced Mediterranean cuisine—and olive oil in dishes that were foreign—to me.

While my mom was bit by the European cuisine bug after

her trip abroad in the sixties when I was nine years old, she didn't serve us nouvelle cuisine like snails and frog legs. I was just a kid, happy with American classics such as soft, white, perfect slices of packaged Wonder Bread spread with peanut butter and jelly and fried chicken cooked in Crisco. (Procter & Gamble developed this popular hydrogenated vegetable shortening that looks like thick white paste. It can be heated higher than lard, but in the twenty-first century I will pass.) So I was in for a new taste bud surprise at the "Mooses"—my godparents' home—when served thick, chewy European breads and eats with more sophisticated flavors than I was used to back at home.

My godmother laughed when I said that I was starving. And then the appetizers were served, little toasts called "bruschetta" drizzled with olive oil. And then, a big bowl of green linguini (we only ate spaghetti) sat next to the veal with herbs. I was mesmerized by the unique green pasta with what my godmother called "pesto sauce"—my first experience with it. It tasted a lot better than macaroni in a box.

Since biblical times, oil, like vinegar, which was known as "the poor man's wine," has played a role in the lives of both the rich, such as royalty, and the poor. In the popular legend of the Four Thieves, the robbers are believed to have used powerful vinegar and herbs to beat getting the deadly plague. But, some olive oil experts believe the savvy foursome used a healing-oil formula. Perhaps they used both oil and vinegar, which together have antiseptic and immunity-boosting properties.

OIL AND VINEGAR

A number of historical reports show that the ancient Babylonians favored oil-and-vinegar dressings. The ancient Egyptians left written accounts of various oil-and-vinegar dressings that included imported herbs and spices.[2]

In the twentieth century, people in the United States were able to purchase prepared dressings that included olive oil and vinegar along with spices and other ingredients. Some of the popular brands of salad dressings we use today go back as far as the early part of that century.

Today, in the twenty-first century, as you know, there are countless olive oils and vinegars on the market. Apple cider and red wine and balsamic vinegars and rice, fruit, and specialty vinegars are all used worldwide. But the fact remains, it's red wine vinegar and apple cider vinegar that seem to get the most credit, and for good reason.

Here, take a look at the two most popular vinegars. Not only were apple cider vinegar and red wine vinegar praised centuries ago, they still deserve praise today. There are many reasons why.

Apple Cider Vinegar and Olive Oil

Researchers are discovering that baby boomers are targets for metabolic syndrome, a cluster of conditions that increase the risk of stroke, diabetes, and heart attack.

Apple cider vinegar may be the perfect and practical modern miracle for baby boomers and seniors (and the younger generations). Metabolic syndrome can be hindered through the use of the simple apple cider vinegar found in your kitchen cupboard or refrigerator.

How? How can this vinegar fight metabolic syndrome? For starters, nutritionists say apple cider vinegar can help you to lose body fat, a culprit that can lead to cholesterol and triglyceride (blood fats) problems, high blood sugar, high blood pressure—all signs of metabolic syndrome.

So, how can apple cider vinegar help you burn fat instead of store it? Ann Louise Gittleman, Ph.D., C.N.S., gave me the plain and simple answer. "Apple cider is a notable fat burner because of its ability to keep sodium and potassium levels balanced. As a potassium-rich food, a couple of ounces of apple cider vinegar a day will put the lid on your appetite because you will be far less hungry and far less bloated."

Apple cider vinegar can help you lose inches faster than pounds, too. "Many individuals boast they shed inches more quickly than they pare pounds. This is again due to the high potassium levels which help to flush out water-logged tissues, created by excessive amounts of water-retaining sodium," adds Gittleman.

Also, organic apple cider vinegar made from fresh apples can contain a healthy dose of pectin. Soluble fiber may help lower "bad" cholesterol by binding with it. Your body then eliminates the fiber, say nutritionists. As a result, you may be able to reduce your risk of heart attack and stroke.

Apple Cider Vinegar, a Dieter's Best Friend

Three-and-one-half ounces of apple cider vinegar contains:

95 percent water
14 calories
0 grams protein
0 grams dietary fiber
0 grams fat
5 grams carbohydrates
6 milligrams calcium
9 milligrams phosphorus
0.6 milligram iron
1 milligram sodium
100 milligrams potassium

22 milligrams magnesium
0.04 milligram copper

(Source: The Healing Powers of Vinegar.)

In addition to adding vinegar to your diet, include olive oil, too. Here, take a look at some vinegar-and-oil weight loss tips:

1. Switch to a salad dressing of vinegar and extra virgin olive oil. One of the biggest sources of fat and calories in the average woman's diet is salad dressing. When you toss a salad of mixed greens, substitute 1 tablespoon each of extra virgin olive oil and vinegar.

2. You lose inches faster when you trim your sandwich, even just a little. Build a more slimming sandwich by substituting poultry for the meat and the cheese; adding plenty of fresh tomatoes, dark green lettuce, and onions; and replacing the mayonnaise with a splash of olive oil and vinegar.

3. Lose the margarine. Giving up margarine and replacing it with olive oil, other healing oils, and a lot of butter will make a big difference, not only in your weight loss, but in your heart health, too.

4. Instead of sautéing your vegetables in margarine, try using olive oil, a splash of vinegar, and another vegetable oil to get a variety of healing benefits.

5. Eating a Mediterranean-style diet—vegetables, fruits, grains, low-fat dairy, fish, and olive oil—can help you shed unwanted weight, but so can getting regular physical activity.

APPLE CIDER VINEGAR FIGHTS
METABOLIC SYNDROME

Disease	How ACV Works
Diabetes	ACV in the diet may help to slow the rise of blood sugar after a high-carbohydrate meal.
Overweight	The fiber in ACV provides bulk and curbs appetite, keeps your sodium–potassium ratio in balance so you're less hungry, and decreases bloating and water retention.
High blood pressure	The potassium in ACV helps reduce hypertension, especially if you team it with potassium-rich fruits and vegetables.
High cholesterol	The insoluble fiber in ACV reduces cholesterol by binding with it. The fiber is then eliminated by the body.

RED WINE VINEGAR AND OLIVE OIL

According to researchers at Harvard University and the National Institute of Aging, resveratrol, an antioxidant found in red wine, inhibited the bad effects of a high-calorie diet in mice and added years to their life span. If people add red wine vinegar (which may contain heart-healthy resveratrol) along with resveratrol-rich foods such as peanuts, blueberries, cranberries, and plums—and olive oil—to their diets, can they stall Father Time?

Yes, it is possible. While apple cider vinegar and olive oil can fight body fat and heart disease, it's the Mediterranean-type red wine and balsamic vinegars teamed with a Mediterranean diet including olive oil that may also fight obesity, which is often linked to heart disease.

Red wine and balsamic vinegars are both derived from grapes. And like red wine, they contain disease-fighting antioxidants such as quercetin and (most likely) resveratrol, especially in the premium, organic brands. While studies have shown that drinking a glass of red wine daily can cut your heart disease risk, consuming these vinegars teamed with olive oil can give you all the same health benefits but without the alcohol. More research is needed to prove that red wine vinegar contains resveratrol. Meanwhile, using it with olive oil on foods that definitely contain resveratrol is a key to fighting metabolic syndrome and stalling age-related diseases.

RED WINE VINEGAR FIGHTS METABOLIC SYNDROME

Disease	How RWV Works
Diabetes	The quercetin in RWV slows the release of insulin.
Heart attack, stroke	The polyphenols in RWV slow down blood clotting by their antioxidant action; the resveratrol (if contained) prevents blood-platelet aggregation and increases HDL cholesterol levels; the tannins reduce platelet aggregation and increase HDL cholesterol levels.

RED WINE VINEGAR FIGHTS METABOLIC SYNDROME (*cont.*)

Disease	How RWV Works
Heart disease	The proanthocyanidins in RWV block the formation of cholesterol deposits on artery walls.
High cholesterol	The catechin in RWV blocks "bad" LDL cholesterol from entering the artery walls, inhibits blood clots from forming, relaxes blood vessels, and inhibits the development of tumors; the flavonoids may help reduce cholesterol levels and prevent the oxidation of LDL cholesterol.

A WEIGHT LOSS SUCCESS STORY

Meet Terry Flores, an Ohio-based, 42-year-old, busy married mom of three boys. One month, I called her and asked her if she wanted to follow my vinegar-based diet plan based on the Mediterranean diet lifestyle. She said that at 5 feet 5 inches and 197 pounds, she was willing to do it.

For two months, she drank a tablespoon of apple cider vinegar in an 8-ounce glass of water three to four times a day. "I also alternated adding red wine vinegar and apple cider vinegar to my meals and salads for flavor. When I cooked my meals with vegetables, fish, and chicken, I always used olive oil. The vegetable oil made it taste heavy, so I only use olive oil now."

While Terry did see almost immediate results, a few times she hit a diet plateau. Therefore, she turned to the Bloat-Busting Meal Plan about every other week. She blames her setbacks on the stress levels in her life, but vows her body responds to the jump-start two-day diet plan.

In two months, Terry lost 17 pounds and four dress sizes. Now at size 12/14, she is confident that she will be wearing a size 10 sooner than later. She says, "My husband and boys keep telling me how great I look. I even like what I see in the mirror again. I know I can do this. After seven years of trying to lose and not being able to, I have hope again."

My Favorite Two-Day "Belly-Busting" Diet

This slimming, healthy meal plan—designed by New Jersey–based nutritionist Toni Gerbino—can help you to lose inches and pare pounds. Also, if you reach that dieter's plateau where the scale numbers won't budge, this is a great way to get back on track.

Breakfast:
Fresh berries (no limit)

Lunch:
4 ounces fresh white meat turkey
Greens with dressing made of fresh parsley, 1 tablespoon each virgin olive oil and apple cider vinegar, and spices to taste
1 cup fresh berries

Dinner:
6 to 8 ounces fresh flounder, sole, or salmon
Asparagus with lemon, apple cider vinegar, and parsley
1 cup fresh berries

Drink a minimum of six 8-ounce glasses of water with fresh lemon throughout the day.

Note: Check with your doctor before starting this or any diet.

15 Diet-Plateau Blasters

These tips are based on the Mediterranean diet and lifestyle, my bible to staying lean and heart healthy.

1. Do eat breakfast every day. It jump-starts your metabolism, provides energy, and staves off hunger pangs to help you stay clear of overeating.

2. Do not eat after 7 P.M. If you must eat something, try a piece of fresh fruit (a fiber-filling apple or pear) and a cup of herbal tea.

3. Forgo foods with trans fats or partially hydrogenated oils (for example, packaged foods such as muffins, cakes, and cookies), which can lead to weight gain.

4. Instead, eat fresh foods (whole grains, fruits, vegetables, fish, legumes, unsalted nuts, and olive oil).

5. Practice portion control. Forget second helpings or eating 6 ounces of fish instead of 3 ounces. Again, read labels. A cup of yogurt is one serving. An orange or apple should be small or medium, not a giant whopper. (Note: If any recipes in this book do not include servings, practice portion control.)

6. When you exercise, up your time by 15 minutes, or increase the intensity if you are doing calorie-burning aerobics.

7. Try working out with weights, which can help boost your metabolism for hours after you are done.

8. On a non-stressful day (or on a stressful one), try a juice-and-vegetable detox diet. It will cleanse your system and allow you more energy and less weight the next day.

9. If you eat white bread, white pasta, or white rice, make the switch to whole grain, which has more filling fiber.

10. Don't get on the scale every day. Building muscle and losing inches is more important than losing pounds. Sooner than later, your body will rebuild itself if you remain true to a healthful diet and exercise.

11. Wear loose-fitting clothing, which will allow you to be more active and comfortable.

12. That spaghetti sauce? It's too high in sodium, which can make you retain water. Dump it, and substitute tomato paste, tomatoes, water, herbs, and spices.

13. Speaking of sodium, potassium-rich fruits and vegetables can help you lose water weight. Make sure you get five to nine servings daily, and drizzle some with olive oil.

14. Watch your sodium intake. Lose the processed foods, canned foods, and lunch meats all of which can contain sodium, which also can raise your blood pressure.

15. Drink six to eight 8-ounce glasses of spring water each day. They will help keep you hydrated, energized, and satisfied.

Pesto Sauce

❖ ❖ ❖

¾ cup Marsala Olive Fruit
   Oil
2 cups fresh basil leaves,
   packed (or arugula)
4 garlic cloves (or to taste)
½ cup fresh parsley, mint,
   or cilantro

¼ cup pine nuts, walnuts,
   macadamia, or nuts of
   your choice
Salt, pepper, and cayenne to
   taste
1 cup Romano cheese,
   grated

Combine olive fruit oil, basil leaves, garlic, parsley, nuts, salt, and pepper in container of a food processor. Process until mixture is coarsely blended. Do not overblend. Transfer mixture into a mixing bowl; stir in cheese. Pesto may be refrigerated and covered with a thin layer of olive oil for several days or when ready to use. Pesto may be frozen very well, but omit cheese. Stir cheese when thawed.

(*Courtesy: Cooking with California Olive Oil: Treasured Family Recipes* by Gemma Sanita Sciabica)

THE GOLDEN SECRETS TO REMEMBER

✓ Oil and vinegar were paired back in ancient history.
✓ In the twentieth century, store-bought dressings teamed oil and vinegar.
✓ Today, in the twenty-first century, health-conscious consumers purchase oil and vinegar separately and marry the foods to keep the result low in sodium, low in calories, and better in quality.

✓ Apple cider vinegar and olive oil can help fight metabolic syndrome, a problem in boomers and seniors that can lead to heart attack, stroke, diabetes, and obesity.

✓ Red wine vinegar and olive oil—with its polyphenol content—can help cut your risk of developing heart disease and obesity.

✓ You can use olive oil to help you jump-start a diet or break a plateau.

CHAPTER 10

The Elixir to
Heart Health

*One tablespoon of olive oil has the power to
wipe out the cholesterol raising effects of two
eggs.*

—Jean Carper[1]

While I did like my godparents' oils and fats, as I reminisced
in the previous chapter, I couldn't help but notice the middle-
aged couple were corpulent (like short olive trees with cracks
and crevices) unlike my lean parents who strived for perfection. During the summertime dinner, we ate at their house outdoors on the patio under an awning to cool the warm air. I
noticed the servings were bigger than smaller. Second helpings went around the wooden table. "More pasta? More bread?"
It was like being at a smorgasbord.

The brown-haired housewife with a full face smiled as I
looked at the big flowers on her colorful muumuu (a flowing

dress ideal for concealing lumps and bumps). I was surprised by the ladles of cream sauces and gobs of butter offered. Everything tasted so good. I enjoyed myself because portion control was something we practiced at home. But I noticed something odd. There was a missing food group on the table.

So back at home the next night in the family room during the heat wave, while eating a slice of watermelon, I asked my mother, "Why don't the Mooses eat fresh vegetables and fruit?" My mom told me that a balance of foods is how to maintain weight. It took a while (years) for me to get it—that you can eat good fats along with good fruits and vegetables. (When I was in my late teens, I cut out fats and starved myself skinny.) It's about finding food balance, and my mother was right.

As the years passed after I graduated from SFSU, I fell into the world of writing nutrition articles. When I was beginning my health career as a diet and nutrition columnist at *Woman's World* magazine, to stay fit, I used olive oil and vinegar on salads with tuna and eggs (in moderation). These simple foods were part of my life because they worked to keep me lean without effort. I also followed a strict but fun regimen of walking to a gym (rain or shine) and working out with free weights to burn off calories and build muscle by using the rowing machine. I didn't want to wear potato sack–type attire like my godmother as I was edging toward "perimenopaws"—a pesky time "when I was morphing into looking like a spayed cat" with a bad attitude.

In addition to keeping you lean and fit, eating heart-healthy foods can also help to cut your risk of developing heart disease. So can eating "good" fats—essential fatty acids. That's what medical doctors will tell you—years ago, today, and most likely in years to come.

In my mid-forties, my blood pressure and cholesterol weren't a big concern. But now, like countless baby boomers and seniors, keeping on top of the numbers game is all too familiar. Now I, like others, face borderline high numbers for cholesterol and blood pressure, thanks to my type-A mom and, as my doctor calls it, my "stressful lifestyle." Sometimes, two dogs, one cat, and two fish aren't enough to keep your cholesterol and blood pressure normal.

Instead of turning to heart medications, I've taken the alternative route. I've upped my exercise (swimming and walking my two dogs), plus you'll find chamomile tea, music, and talking to friends on my daily agenda. But trying to win the battle against the potential for developing heart disease, especially as an aging boomer who also now has less estrogen, is a challenge.

But the good news is, olive oil may be a heart-healthy companion to put in the arsenal against heart disease. In fact, researchers for the U.S. Food and Drug Administration believe olive oil can lower your risk for developing heart disease.

THE "GOOD" FATS

Several years ago, when I interviewed Dr. Artemis P. Simopoulos, author of *The Omega Diet* (HarperCollins, 1998), she told me that there are two kinds of essential fats (EFAs), omega-6 and omega-3. The problem: The American diet contains more omega-6 fatty acids (found in foods such as mayonnaise and salad dressing) than omega-3s. This imbalance makes us more prone to heart disease.

At the time, I wasn't excited about this information, nor did I truly understand it. Today, I realize that this doctor knew what she was talking about, and now I get it. Perhaps, I'm more interested because of the age thing. I realize that if I don't find the delicate balance of EFAs, I may end up taking prescription heart medications, or worse.

SuperFoods Rx author Steven Pratt, M.D., notes in his book that the best balance of omega-6 to omega-3 is somewhere between 1 to 1 and 4 to 1. "Unfortunately, the typical Western diet contains fourteen to twenty-five times more omega-6 than omega-3 fatty acids," he notes. "Too much omega-6 (the oil that dominates our typical diet) promotes an inflammatory state, which in turn increases your risk for blood clots and narrowing of blood vessels."[2]

But the consensus is that the jury is still out about how much omega-3 versus omega-6 you should incorporate in your daily menu. Olive oil, a "good," monounsaturated fat, contains both omega-3 and omega-6 fatty acids.

Dr. Simopoulos offered hope. She told me that we can eat foods that contain the "good" essential fatty acids such as omega-3—found in eggs, fish, and olive oil—along with vegetables, fruits, and legumes. Eating these foods, as do heart healthy people who follow the Mediterranean diet, whether in the European countries or in America, can protect the heart by raising the antioxidant levels, reducing the risk of blood clots, and normalizing blood pressure and heartbeat. Countless people around the world, like you and me, can do the same—begin to balance the EFAs in our diet.

The following heart-healthy tips are from Dr. Simopoulos. Her advice, which I included in my book *Doctors' Orders*, was on target because these helpful hints back up the Mediterranean diet. But adding saturated fat and other healing oils—in moderation—is gaining acceptance by medical researchers and people around the world.

- *Enrich your diet with omega-3 fatty acids.* Eat fatty fish, such as salmon two or more times a week.
- *Use olive oil as your primary oil.*
- *Eat nine or more servings of fruits and vegetables daily.* People in the Mediterranean countries consume plenty of fresh produce, and have enjoyed good health due to the disease-fighting antioxidant benefits.
- *Eat more peas, beans, and nuts.* They are free of saturated fat and cholesterol.
- *Use sparingly oils high in the omega-6 fatty acids.* These include corn oil, safflower oil, peanut oil, soybean oil, sunflower seed oil, cottonseed oil and mayonnaise. These cooking oils do have some health merits, as shown in Chapter 8.
- *Avoid trans fatty acids.* If you see "partially hydrogenated" on a food label, forgo the product. These substances are often found in baked goods and snack foods.

Olive Oil and Blood Pressure

For years, I've been writing about the Mediterranean diet, as well as abiding by it myself. In a nutshell, you can have your fat and lower your blood pressure, too, if you eat like they do in Greece and southern Italy, according to medical experts. For instance, if you replace some of the saturated fat, like butter and cheese, in your diet with extra virgin olive oil, you may be able to lower your blood pressure or even cut down on your blood pressure medicine or stop taking it altogether, according to the editors of *The Folk Remedy Encyclopedia*.[3]

The editors add, "But according to the American Institute

of Cancer Research olive oil is only a small part of healthy eating in that part of the world." Again, it's the combination of eating little red meat and processed foods, eating more fish and vegetables, and drinking a little red wine that makes the diet healthful—not just one ingredient. It's the total diet and lifestyle package that may help keep blood pressure numbers normal—not just olive oil.[4]

Research shows, too, that a Mediterranean diet, which is similar to the Dietary Approaches to Stop Hypertension (DASH) diet, is linked with both systolic (the top number, which describes the heart's force) and diastolic (the bottom number, which describes the tension between the heartbeats) blood pressure. Olive oil may make as much of a difference as fruits and vegetables in getting a grip on the blood pressure.

And chances are, if you have high blood pressure, you may have high cholesterol, too.

OLIVE OIL AND CHOLESTEROL

Did you know that saturated and trans fats are unhealthy culprits in high blood cholesterol? In adults, total cholesterol levels of 240 milligrams per deciliter or higher are considered high risk, and levels from 200 to 239 milligrams per deciliter are considered borderline high risk, according to the AHA.

A middle-aged married couple in Osterville, Massachusetts, told me they are devout users of olive oil—and it seems they are reaping the rewards. C. L. Fornari, aka "The Garden Lady," says, "Both my husband and I have high levels of HDL or 'good' cholesterol, and we are convinced that the amount of olive oil we eat is a major reason for those high levels of HDL." And yes, Fornari is aware that olive oil is rich in disease-fighting polyphenols, which are believed to help control cholesterol levels and lower the risk of heart disease. She adds, "Dan and I use the freshest, full-flavored oils for salads and bread. We use other cold-pressed, virgin oil for cooking."

Research proves that polyphenols can help you stay heart-healthy. A study was done on olive oil and its effects on the hearts of 200 healthy men between the ages of 20 and 60 at six centers in Spain, Denmark, Finland, Italy, and Germany. In a three-week period, the men took a tablespoon of three different olive oils (they varied in phenolic content). The findings: All three of the olive oils raised the "good" cholesterol, lowered the total cholesterol, and lowered triglycerides. The results proved that the polyphenols in the monounsaturated fatty acid benefits the HDL cholesterol and may lower the risk of developing other heart problems.[5]

OLIVE OIL AND BLOOD SUGAR

So, if olive oil can help reduce the risk of developing heart disease, what can it do about diabetes, especially type 2 diabetes (the non-insulin type that can be controlled with lifestyle changes and, if necessary, medication)? Yes, the liquid gold comes to the rescue again.

Studies show that olive oil as used in the Mediterranean diet may help reduce the risk of developing metabolic syndrome—a cluster of conditions that increase the odds of heart attacks, stroke, and diabetes—which is becoming all too common in baby boomers. If you have high blood sugar, this is a sign that you may have type 2 diabetes.

A study was conducted at a university hospital in Italy. People with metabolic syndrome (99 men and 81 women) followed a Mediterranean-style diet and were taught how to increase their daily intake of whole grains, fruits, vegetables, nuts, and olive oil.

The results: In two years, researchers found that the Mediterranean diet group lowered their weight, blood pressure, total cholesterol (while boosting their "good" HDL cholesterol), triglycerides, glucose, and insulin. The authors believe that the Mediterranean-style diet might be a key in fighting metabolic syndrome, an age-related problem that is hitting home in America for both boomers and seniors.[6]

The AHA recommends:

- Further reducing trans fatty acids in the diet
- Minimizing intake of food and beverages with added sugars
- Emphasizing physical activity and weight control
- Eating a diet rich in vegetables, fruits, and whole-grain foods
- Avoiding tobacco
- Achieving and maintaining healthy cholesterol, blood pressure, and glucose levels

TAKE FATS TO HEART

Trans fats are a hot topic because these hydrogenated fats found in processed foods can be harmful to your heart. According to the AHA, some researchers believe they raise cholesterol levels more than saturated fats do. Plus, trans fats also can up "bad" LDL cholesterol and lower "good" HDL cholesterol when used instead of healthy oils such as olive oil. By switching to heart-healthy oils, you may lower your risk of developing heart disease—high blood pressure, high cholesterol, and diabetes.

The AHA recommends that you:

- Limit your intake of saturated fat to less than 7 percent of your total calories if you are healthy and over the age of 2
- Limit your trans fat to less than 1 percent of your total calories
- Limit your total fat intake to 25 to 35 percent of your total calories
- Get your remaining fat intake from sources of monounsaturated and polyunsaturated fats such as vegetable oils, nuts, seeds, and fish

In addition, did you know that your dentist may be able to predict if you are prone to heart disease? Poor dental hygiene, according to medical experts, can be linked to cardiovascular disease, strokes, and infections. So, while you put olive oil in your daily menu, don't forget to keep your regular dental appointments, too.

As baby boomers and seniors cope with keeping their cholesterol, blood pressure, triglycerides, and blood sugar levels in check, let's take a look at olive oil and its promise to help you lose unwanted body fat and maintain your weight.

Asparagus and Wild Mushroom Pappardelle

❖ ❖ ❖

This hearty fresh pasta dish takes only about 25 minutes to prepare. Wine suggestion: a sauvignon blanc with herbal nuances, preferably a medium-bodied one to balance the oil and cheese.

8 to 12 ounces fresh pap-
pardelle pasta
3 tablespoons The Olive
Press Arbequina extra
virgin olive oil
½ bunch asparagus, cut into
1-inch lengths
½ large onion, halved and
sliced
¼ pound wild or cultivated
mushrooms, cleaned and
cut into bite-size pieces

Salt and freshly ground
pepper to taste
¾ cup dry white wine
2 tomatoes, chopped
2 tablespoons chopped
Italian parsley
2 tablespoons freshly grated
Parmesan
Truffle oil
The Olive Press Arbequina
extra virgin olive oil, to
drizzle

Bring a large pot of salted water to a boil for the pasta.
Begin cooking the pasta about 5 minutes before the sauce is
ready. Preheat a large sauté pan. Add the olive oil and then
the asparagus. Cook approximately 1 minute. Add the onion
and the mushrooms and cook an additional minute. Season
with salt and pepper. Deglaze with the wine and reduce by
half, about 5 minutes. Remove from the heat and stir in
chopped tomatoes. Drain the cooked pasta and add it to the
sauce. Add the parsley and toss lightly. Check seasoning and
adjust as needed. Divide the pasta among serving bowls, top
with the Parmesan, and drizzle with truffle oil or extra virgin
olive oil. Serves 4.

*Fresh pappardelle is available packaged and freshly cut
in upscale markets and specialty pasta shops.

(*Courtesy:* The Olive Press)

THE GOLDEN SECRETS TO REMEMBER

✓ Finding a delicate balance of omega-3s and omega-6s can help you prevent heart disease.

✓ Incorporate more omega-3s—eggs, fish, and olive oil—into your diet to get your essential fatty acids.

✓ Stay clear of oils high in omega-6s—such as salad dressing and mayonnaise. Opt for red wine vinegar and olive oil.

✓ While olive oil may help to lower your blood pressure, don't forget to lose the processed foods and add fish and vegetables to your diet menu.

✓ If your LDL cholesterol is 100 milligrams per deciliter or greater, lower your eating plan to 25 to 35 percent calories from fat. Monitor your saturated fat and dietary cholesterol intake.

✓ To prevent or control type 2 diabetes, cut saturated fats and foods with added sugars from your diet. Plus, focus on regular exercise, and keep your weight in check.

✓ Stay clear of artery-clogging trans fats, found in processed and fried foods. (Read the product label or ask the fast-food chain what type of oil they use.)

11

The Olive Oil Diet

*There's probably no food choice you'll make
that does more for your health and weight loss
efforts than olive oil.*

—Connie Peraglier, R.D.[1]

Several years ago, during the winter when our ski resort town was blanketed in snow, I paid a visit to the office of the *Tahoe Daily Tribune* in South Lake Tahoe. I was there to meet the editor and get my photo taken. I was the new weekly food columnist. When the editor greeted me, she commented about how lanky I was. (I smiled because it's been said people don't believe a lean chef can cook. But in defense of all the skinny chefs, it takes work and know-how to stay lean like my favorite dog breed: the Brittany.) The food column was almost called "The Skinny Cook"!

As the years have passed, I confess at times it's still a struggle to maintain a size 4 and pull on skinny jeans, especially when I'm in the kitchen testing dishes. I must test, which makes me think I'm like an olive tree or golden goose that doesn't want to be uprooted or stuffed. I cook and bake dishes for readers that serve four; I'm solo. That single status reminds me of one winter when I finished eating two slices of fresh holiday apple-cranberry pie (with nut oil and butter that's supposed to fill you up, not out). Clad in sweatpants and a sweatshirt, I thought, "I look like my godmother, Mrs. Moose."

Ironically, that night I watched *Julie and Julia*—one of my favorite films. I love the scene when blogger Julie Powell aims to whip up more than 500 recipes from Julia Child's cookbook *Mastering the Art of French Cooking* in one year, and in one scene she complained that she felt fat, like I do when testing my dishes for articles and the Healing Powers series. I thank freezer inventor and scientist Carl von Linde; my sibling, a self-professed food critic; and my dear fur children who love anything I create in the kitchen.

As a food and health author, I walk the line of maintaining an ideal weight. It's a juggling act to stay lean. I received gourmet chocolate on my doorstop every week, for instance, when I wrote *The Healing Powers of Chocolate*. It's a challenge to balance the scales when healthful foods like healing oils still contain fat and calories. Olive oil (despite its 120 calories per tablespoon) plays a role on days like these. My mother taught me about balance. I eat less than more to make up for overindulging. So I survive on skinny foods (fruits, vegetables, nuts, and oils) on the "semi" Paleo Diet, my hunter and gatherer mode, like the way people ate thousands of years ago.

People with high blood pressure and high cholesterol sometimes struggle with tipping the scale—but not always. You can be at your ideal weight and yet have blood pressure higher than 120/80. Blame it on your genes (or the demanding dog, wife, husband, or boss), which can play a role in heart disease, and obesity, too.

If you're overweight, keep in mind body fat can attract heart-related diseases like a magnet. The good news is, olive oil may help you to take it off.

Eric Armstrong of Mountain View, California, vows that olive oil helps him stave off hunger pangs and boosts his energy—two keys to maintaining your ideal weight.

"I found that building a diet around olive oil helped to suppress hunger and increase energy. Taking it by itself was most effective, but I found it difficult to digest—so I began dipping my bread in it, along with vinegar, as is the custom in Europe. I also put a couple of tablespoons on my cereal in the morning, as part of a dairy-free milk substitute I make myself. It definitely adds to my energy throughout the day," he says.

Drizzling olive oil on a salad, sandwich, stir-fry, or vegetables makes you feel satisfied and full—two secrets to maintaining a healthy weight effortlessly. A study that proves the proof is in the oil has shown how natural oils and fats regulate sensation of feeling full after eating, with olive oil leading the way. Work groups at the University of Vienna studied four different dietary fats and oil: lard, butterfat, rapeseed oil, and olive oil. After three months, olive oil proved to be the blue ribbon winner, with thanks to its aroma producing the most satiety—that is, what can help you feel full and not want to overeat.[2]

Smelling the aroma of olive oil may help you feel full, too. A report published in the *American Journal of Clinical Nutrition* said so. In a study of 11 men, some ate plain low-fat yogurt, and others ate yogurt that included olive extract. It was the scent of the oil that provided satiety reported the scientists at the German Research Center for Food Chemistry.[3]

Indeed, olive oil can suppress your appetite, and perhaps

it does just that in Italian-style meals, which include dipping bread into olive oil before beginning the entrée. Keep in mind, however, that while extra virgin olive oil is rich in good-for-you polyphenols, too much of anything can be bad. And yes, that includes olive oil. Remember, it has calories—120 per tablespoon and 14 whopping grams of fat. But, that doesn't stop some people from indulging in the liquid gold by the tablespoon straight from the bottle on a daily basis to lose pounds.

FROM OLIVE OIL TO SHANGRI-LA

Meet Dr. Seth Roberts. Several years ago, he pondered why most diets fail. He decided to be a human rat and used sugar water and extra light olive oil to drop unwanted pounds. When I interviewed the soft-spoken man, he discussed his weight-loss antics.

Back in 2000, Roberts decided to diet because he wanted to be thinner for his 5 foot 11 inch frame. It took him about three months to lose 40 pounds by incorporating fructose water into his diet. He claims that weight is regulated by a "set point." If your weight is below your set point, hunger sets in and you'll want to eat more to feel more satisfied. Roberts believes you can tweak that set point by eating a food that is without flavor—you'll eat less. In fact, Dr. Roberts ended up writing a bestseller, *The Shangri-La Diet: The No Hunger Eat Anything Weight-Loss Plan* (Putnam, 2006) about his experience.

Later, he used extra light olive oil to maintain his weight loss. The idea to take a tablespoon of olive oil—light or not— is a bit hard for me to swallow. But the good professor of psychology at the University of California at Berkeley assured me that it isn't bad at all.

In his book, he writes that a friend told him about "a type of olive, called extra-light" that is bland—no flavor. He notes, "My friend understood that my theory predicted that the most potent weight-loss foods provided calories without flavor. Fructose water did this because of a special wrinkle: sweetness didn't count. ELOO was another way. According to my theory, 100 calories of ELOO should have the same effect as the 100 calories of fructose water."[4]

And it did. But the extra light olive oil also "took less time," according to Dr. Roberts. "No preparation was needed, unlike sugar water." So, it's this olive oil taken daily—just a few spoonfuls daily—that helped the doctor maintain his weight loss. At 5 feet 11 inches, he had lost 40 pounds; and these days, he admitted, he has maintained his weight of a 30-pound weight loss—170 pounds—and gives credit to both the fructose water and the olive oil. "For a few years, I drank only ELOO and didn't use fructose water," he writes. Then, he added the fructose water back in because "it is pleasant."[5]

Also, during our first interview, he told me (and he writes in his book) that he continues to use both—extra light olive oil or some other flavorless oil at home, sucrose water when he's away from home. He doesn't use measured amounts either. If he has packed on a few pounds, he will drink more. If he is too "thin," he will drink less.

These days, Roberts is experimenting once again, and this time it's with walnut oil (1 tablespoon) and flaxseed oil (2 tablespoons) daily. "I am still trying to determine the optimum type and amount of oil but I am sure I will continue forever because of the weight and health benefits."

Speaking of different diets, as a former diet and nutrition

columnist for *Woman's World* magazine, I used to write about every diet imaginable, from the cabbage soup diet to high-protein diets.

EAT FAT TO LOSE FAT

It's funny, but as I wrote about paring pounds, I continued to eat the Mediterranean diet type of foods—vegetables, fruits, whole grains, even pizza—and I maintained my 122 pounds through it all. Despite the fact that I didn't have a weight problem, I once again was faced with progressive medical doctors discussing "good" fats with me.

I interviewed Dr. Barry Sears, for example, who wrote *Enter the Zone.* He told me that it was important to add the right amount of fat to your diet. Yes, fat!

"I know it's shocking," Dr. Sears said, "but you have to eat fat in order to lose fat. You have to stop thinking of food in terms of calories and fat grams alone and start thinking of it as a mechanism for controlling the flow of hormones."

The fact is, fats and proteins trigger the release of hormones that neutralize the effect of insulin released by carbohydrates. So, adding more fat and protein to your diet means you'll actually store less fat.

But you don't want to load up on saturated fat, the artery-clogging fat found mainly in animal products. You want to avoid overindulging in these fats because they tend to raise insulin levels, which will defeat your fat-burning goal. In Chapter 8, "More Healing Oils," I discuss the oils that are good for you in moderation. It's these same oils that can help you to fight fat forever.

I also interviewed nutritionists Gene and Joyce Daoust, who taught me about "good" fats, too. They told me unsaturated fat (vegetable oils like safflower oil, sunflower oil, and corn oil) and monounsaturated fat (olive oil, canola oil, olives, macadamia nuts, and avocados) are good for you and can help you to burn fat.

Here are some important facts I learned about eating "good" fat:

- It boosts your energy.
- It triggers the release of CCK, a hormone that signals your brain that you're full and should stop eating.
- It contains fat-soluble compounds to help metabolize fat-soluble vitamins A, D, E, and K.
- It contains omega-3 and omega-6 fatty acids (found in fatty fishes, such as tuna), which are essential for fat metabolism.
- It helps slow down the rate of carbohydrate absorption into the bloodstream and helps to lower the rate of insulin secretion.

USE YOUR FAT BUDGET

So, we do need some fat. The consensus is to consume about 40 to 60 grams per day. Also, do not deprive yourself of good-for-you fatty foods—some with olive oil, others without.

Favorite Food	"Good" Fats	Fat Grams
Pizza	Order vegetable toppings, and hold the meat and extra cheese; drizzle olive oil on top; and order a dark green side salad with vegetables.	5 grams per slice

Favorite Food	"Good" Fats	Fat Grams
Peanut butter	A rich spread high in fat, but it's mainly monounsaturated and polyunsaturated fats, which are healthier for your heart than saturated fat.	8 grams per tablespoon
Eggs	Even though egg yolks contain fat, they also contain vit-amins A, B, D, and E.	6 grams per egg
Avocados	High in fat, but most of it is mono-unsaturated, which tends to improve cholesterol and protect rather than clog arteries.	8 grams per fruit
Almonds	"Almonds are probably the best all-around nut. Most of the fats of the almond are poly-unsaturated and high in linoleic acid, our main essential oil," notes Elson Haas, M.D., author of *Staying Healthy with Nutrition* (Celestial Arts, 2006).	5.4 grams per 10 nuts

THE SKINNY ON TRANS FATS

The good news is that "trans fats" is becoming a household word. You can pick up a food item and read the label to see if it contains trans fats—those bad-for-you partially hydrogenated vegetable oils found in packaged, processed foods. It's lurking inside such items as pastries, pies, cookies, cakes, muffins, margarine, and vegetable shortening. In fact, the U.S. Food and Drug Administration is considering regulating trans fats because they're unhealthy.

And thanks to the FDA guidelines of January 1, 2006, the labeling of foods includes the amount of trans fats in each product. The glitch is that food manufacturers are hesitant to stop using trans fats, since this ingredient is less costly than healthier oils such as olive oil—and it helps preserve products' shelf life. Worse, many of these fatty foods containing these fats claim to be trans fat–free.

A good way to decode foods for their trans fat content is to check the ingredients list. If you see the words "partially hydrogenated oils," "hydrogenated oils," or "vegetable shortening," stay clear. These are red flags and—nice words for a "bad" fat.

This can get tricky. For instance, I purchased a box of dark chocolate brownie mix. I wanted to add olive oil to see if it worked and tasted good. The food label read, "Trans fat 0 g," but it also included the words "partially hydrogenated soybean and/or cottonseed oil."

Confused and hesitant to bake my healthful brownies, I contacted Marisa Moore, R.D., American Dietetic Association spokesperson based in Atlanta, Georgia. She told me, "According to the US Food and Drug Administration (FDA) guidelines, trans fat does not have to be listed if the total fat in a product is less than 0.5 grams per serving and no claims are made about fat, fatty acids and cholesterol content."

In addition, Moore says, "If trans fats per serving equals 0.5 grams or less, manufacturers are allowed to list the trans fat as 0 (zero) on the label. Therefore, you may find products that list 0 grams trans fat on the label, while 'partially hydrogenated vegetable oil' appears in the ingredient list."

Rather than play the game of seeing how far down the list of ingredients trans fats may be, it's safer to change your game plan of buying food and cooking it. Read: Make homemade brownies or use a product that doesn't contain partially hydrogenated oil.The best advice: If you follow the Mediterranean Diet—vegetables, fruits, grains, fish, legumes, and olive oil—you won't have to decipher packaged goods. You will be eating fresh foods, and this will help you to fight fat, and to lower your risk of developing age-related diseases that are linked to body fat, too.

An easy-to-remember rule is: Limit your intake of trans fats to no more than 1 percent of your total calories. On a 2,000-calorie diet, that equals 2 grams per day. "It's important to seek products that are trans fat free and also low in saturated fat," says Moore. That way, you can achieve a trim, healthy body.

NEVER DIET AGAIN

You really don't have to deprive yourself to lose pounds or maintain your weight. It's all about incorporating healthful eating habits into your lifestyle. For instance, when I go to a sandwich outlet, I order whole wheat bread, extra tomatoes, lettuce, green bell peppers, one piece of swiss chesse, olive oil, and vinegar. And now, I also ask for avocado and olives.

Speaking of olives . . . Recently, I ordered a vegetarian pizza. Usually, I order the normal tomato sauce, spinach, and mushrooms. This time, however, I overheard the man who took my order say "basil" and "olive oil." I quickly inquired, since I had no clue they offered a pesto sauce with these two items. So, I ordered the green sauce with spinach, tomatoes, and olives. Do you see how you can treat yourself to full-fat foods and still eat healthy as well as not pack on unwanted pounds? What's more, if time allows, you can whip up your own pizza and use pesto sauce.

Fresh Fig Appetizer

❖ ❖ ❖

8 fresh figs
Grated peel of 1 lemon or orange
8 teaspoons ricotta or goat cheese (low fat)
2 tablespoons honey or pure maple syrup

1/8 teaspoon almond extract
1/3 cup pistachios or cashews, ground
1/4 cup Marsala Olive Oil or 1/4 cup extra virgin lavender olive oil

Remove stems, halve figs lengthwise, and place on serving plate. In a mixing bowl, stir together peel, ricotta, honey, and almond extract. Place one teaspoon of ricotta mixture on each half of fig. Sprinkle with nuts, drizzle with olive oil, and served chilled.

Note: Figs may be dipped 1/3 from bottom in melted dark chocolate. Place on waxed paper lined sheet to firm up.

(*Courtesy: Cooking with California Olive Oil: Recipes from the Heart for the Heart* by Gemma Sanita Sciabica)

Once you realize that you can eat food and have your pizza, too, you'll get a handle on your weight. But then, while maintaining your ideal weight, there's the aging factor, which affects more than body fat and pounds. In the next chapter, I will discuss why olive oil is getting a good reputation around the world for turning back the clock.

Grilled Chicken on Country Bread

❖ ❖ ❖

¼ cup olive oil or extra virgin olive oil, divided
2 tablespoons Dijon mustard
2 tablespoons balsamic vinegar
2 to 3 teaspoons chopped fresh tarragon or 1 teaspoon dried tarragon
½ teaspoon salt
4 boneless skinless chicken breasts (about 1½ pounds)
8 slices crusty country-style bread, lightly toasted if desired
¼ cup mayonnaise*
¾ medium avocado, sliced
2 large Roma tomatoes, sliced
4 leaves of lettuce

Combine 2 tablespoons olive oil, mustard, vinegar, tarragon, and salt in sealable large food storage bag or shallow dish; mix lightly to blend. Add chicken breasts; turn to coat and marinate at least 20 minutes. (For more intense flavor, marinate chicken longer in the refrigerator.)

Heat remaining 2 tablespoons olive oil in medium skillet over medium heat. Remove chicken from marinade; place in skillet. Cook, covered, 7 to 8 minutes per side or until internal temperature of chicken is 170°. Add 2 to 3 tablespoons water, if needed, to prevent marinade from overbrowning. Remove from heat.

Spread one side of each bread with mayonnaise. Top with chicken, avocado, tomato, and lettuce. Serves 4.

Note: Chicken breasts can be sliced or shredded after removed from heat. Serve with marinated green olives. Mayonnaise variations: For tarragon mayonnaise, blend additional chopped tarragon and a dash of salt into mayonnaise. For Dijon mayonnaise, blend 1 teaspoon Dijon mustard into mayonnaise.

(*Courtesy:* North American Olive Oil Association)

THE GOLDEN SECRETS TO REMEMBER

✓ Olive oil can help to suppress your appetite. Go ahead—drizzle it on bread the way Europeans do before a meal . . .

✓ . . . But don't overdo a good thing. Olive oil is a fat and does have 120 calories per tablespoon.

✓ Extra light olive oil, which is without flavor, may help you to maintain your weight, or "set point."

✓ Eating "good" fats can give you energy, stop you from overeating, help your body metabolize the fat-soluble vitamins, and provide essential fatty acids.

✓ Savor a moderate amount of fatty foods such as pizza and eggs because these favorites contain "good" fats and other nutrients.

✓ Learn how to decode the ingredients lists of food products, which often call trans fats "partially hydrogenated oils," "hydrogenated oils," or "vegetable oils." Then run, not walk, away from these foods.

✓ To get a trim body, limit your intake of trans fats to no more than 1 percent of your total calories.

1 2

Antiaging Wonder Food

*Italians . . . seemed to never die. They eat olive
oil all day long . . . and that's what does it.*
—William Kennedy[1]

Not unlike Julie Powell in *Julie and Julia,* I, too, was influenced by a woman with a love of food and Europe. In my forties, on a balmy spring night, typical of the San Francisco Bay Area peninsula, I was sitting inside an air-conditioned authentic Italian restaurant with Virginia, a cultured octogenarian. As her devoted confidante during the first course to last course of a decadent meal, I listened to her tales of yesteryear (in between sipping tea and indulging in olive oil).

That special evening, my friend, a retired musician, told me about her love affair with a maestro from Brussels. They had played in symphonies more than a dozen times in different European countries. She spoke of romance and European cuisine interchangeably. Like an ancient olive tree producing olives for healing olive oil, she continued to give gifts to people that helped their bodies, minds, and spirits.

I was not a foodie (watching my weight makes living to

eat not an option), so I learned that night to savor French bread dipped in olive oil and to enjoy a large salad with vegetables drizzled with oil and red wine vinegar. Virginia, who appeared to be in her seventies (and lived to almost 100), sipped red wine and encouraged me to eat good fatty foods (from olive oil to chocolate) to stay young and healthy. (I did eat but like a cavewoman.) It was nights, like that one, with my surrogate grandmother, that I believed in a food-love connection. Eating good food can feed the soul and enhance good health and longevity.

Years later, living in the Sierra, one morning after I finished my breakfast of fruit and oatmeal, I pondered, "Why is Japan, not Greece, ranked number-one for longevity?" I quickly called my go-to person, *The Omega Diet* author Artemis P. Simopoulos, M.D., and asked her, "Why aren't the Europeans ranked as having the longest life span? What about the Mediterranean diet?"

She told me that the Cretes did have the longest life span, as well as the lowest rates of heart disease and cancer, thanks to eating antioxidant-rich foods. But lately, they have been replacing these good foods with the high-fat and processed foods of the Western diet, much like the traditional Hawaiians, whom I wrote about several years ago. Fast food is cheaper and faster, but the numbers show that eating it also leads to a shorter life.

Other nutritionists and medical doctors agree. People in the European countries as well as in America are spending less time cooking in the kitchen and more time eating at fast-food chains and restaurants, which boast unhealthy fats. Still, on the upside, more chefs and food outlets know that Mediterranean fare is healthy and so are offering the antioxidant-rich antiaging foods, including heart-healthy oils such as canola and olive oil.

CAN OLIVE OIL TURN BACK THE CLOCK?

Recently, I took one of those online "Real Age" tests online. Since I've been tagged a health and fitness expert, you would think that I'd pass the self-quiz with flying colors, right? Well, not exactly. My real age was 57, which was 3.9 years less than my calendar age of 61. While I wasn't thrilled, I realized it could be worse (because I love boundless energy and feel 40, and am still in the healthy tier one ranking via my health insurance company).

To me, the test results seemed confusing. But I got a second opinion from Marisa Moore, R.D, American Dietetic Association spokesperson. She gave me the low-down on my dietary needs, based upon my test evaluation and recommendations. It's as easy as 1-2-3.

1 **More Vitamin E:** The test results suggested I up my intake of vitamin E. Moore says, "Based on the Dietary Reference Intakes (DRIs), healthy adult women and men should aim for 15 mg vitamin E per day. The recommendation is the same for males and females greater than 14 years old." Your best food sources are walnut oil, soybean oil, olive oil, peanut butter, and wheat germ.

2 **More Essential Fatty Acids:** Then, the test analysis hit me in the belly because I prefer to be a vegetarian— a strict one most of the time. It was recommended that I add fish or other sources of omega-3 fatty acids to my diet at least several times a week.

Moore says, "Aim for 1–2grams of omega-3 fatty acids per day. This is ideal to help reduce LDL (bad) cholesterol and to help with brain development. It's best to get your omega-3s from food." So, again, I now have albacore tuna in my pantry; I also purchase fresh salmon. But, I confess I don't like fish as much as I did as a kid. Also, those little signs about mercury toxins that stare at me while I stand in line to purchase fresh fish at the supermarket are a bit scary. The omega-3s are found in more than just salmon and tuna.

"Omega-3 fatty acids are polyunsaturated fats found mostly in seafood. Good sources include fatty, cold-water fish such as mackerel, halibut and herring. Flax-seeds, flax oil and walnuts also contain omega-3 fatty acids, and small amounts are found in soybean and canola oils. They have a protective effect by reducing blood clot formation, reducing triglyceride levels and may be important in your diet to help prevent cardio-vascular disease. Aim for 2 servings of fish per week," explains Moore.

Flaxseed oil is on my must-try list. Walnuts I can do.

3   **More Unsaturated Fat:** The test results also noted that I should eat more unsaturated fat without increasing my consumption of saturated fat. Worse, because I evidently am eating less than the average amount of unsaturated fats, my biological age may be slightly older. "How could this be?" I pondered. "I am an olive oil book author."

Moore says, "Olive oil is a way to increase your intake of heart healthy fats. You can also use olive oil to make salad dressings, drizzle on grilled or roasted vegetables, in marinades and sautés." Plus, she adds, "Olive oil is a great source of monounsaturated fats while soybean and corn oil are polyunsaturated fats. Both fats may help lower your blood cholesterol when used in place of saturated fats in your diet." Ironically, I know this now, but I guess it's a task to practice what you preach.

I had thought that my borderline high cholesterol was due to genes, not my diet. It's true, I have eaten those big, sugar bran and pumpkin muffins and extra large bagels from bakeries—which use unhealthy fats. This test—and Moore's personal comments—taught me that while I thought I was on the "good"-fats track, there is more I can do—starting with incorporating olive oil, vitamin E, and fish in my daily diet. But that's not all . . .

Olive oil can be beneficial for people of all ages including the elderly. Spanish researchers evaluated the effect of adding olive oil to the diets of healthy elderly people. The results: Extra virgin olive oil reduced total cholesterol, and also increased HDL "good" cholesterol.[2]

THE FOUNTAIN OF OIL AND VINEGAR

I often tout the antiaging potential of both red wine and balsamic vinegars. Why? Researchers I interviewed several years ago said there's a possibility that vinegar contains resveratrol just like heart-healthy red wine and grape juice. Well, in 1999 *and* 2006, Dr. LeRoy Creasy analyzed a cheap red wine vinegar, and both times, he claims, he didn't find any resveratrol. But the question remains, if he used a high-quality vinegar, would it make a difference?

Still, even if red wine and balsamic vinegars contain only disease-fighting polyphenols (and we know they do), some foods such as blueberries, plums, peanuts, and red wine—all part of the Mediterranean diet—do indeed contain resveratrol.

So, teaming these antiaging foods with olive oil may help people around the globe—not just in the Mediterranean basin—to lose body fat and stall age-related diseases. These resveratrol-rich foods combined with other nutrient-rich "superfoods" that contain other disease-fighting compounds can help people fight the aging process and live a longer, healthier life.

Speaking of turning back the clock, I started noticing articles online about challenges of aging. Now, I wrote about all of those topics in my book *Doctors' Orders*. However, when I am hit with Real Age test results and told I need to pay higher health insurance rates, you can bet that I'm going to get my aging woes in a row.

DEFYING AGING WITH OLIVE OIL

Arthritis

The Aging Factor: As we age, our joints begin to degenerate. According to the Arthritis Foundation, osteoarthritis affects nearly 21 million Americans, mostly after age 45; women are more commonly affected than men.

It's Personal: In my sixties, I don't have arthritis yet, but I know people who do have aches and pains. While a heating pad does the trick for me after I shovel snow or overdo it on the bike or using hand weights, it doesn't mean that I am immune to arthritis woes. A friend of mine who is my age does have arthritis, in her hip. A neighbor who is in his seventies has osteoarthritis and is bedridden. And, I can't forget how my late beloved Brittany, Dylan, suffered from arthritis—a problem I never thought would affect a 40-pound dog. But to watch him not be able to jump up into the car or onto the bed was enough to make me see how stiff joints are not fun.

Olive Oil + Rx: While olive oil can be beneficial, omega-3 oils are also important for the lubrication of joints. They reduce prostaglandins. Also, rheumatologists will tell you that staying physically active (like recommended in the Mediterranean lifestyle) is another way to shake the pain of stiff joints.

Cancer

The Aging Factor: The longer we live, the greater are our odds of facing cancer—when free radical molecules in the body cause normal cells to grow and divide in an out-of-control manner.

It's Personal: The big C is frightening to everyone (at any age). My father died of liver cancer. As a DES daughter (DES is a synthetic estrogen that was given to about 4.8 million women in the United States between 1938 and 1971, and has been linked to a rare from of cancer in their daughters and sons), when I have regular Pap smears, I can't forget that I am at a higher risk for developing cervical cancer. Again, as we age, cancer becomes a more likely scenario, whether it is skin cancer or breast cancer—it can affect all of us. Nobody is immune—not me, you, or even our pets.

Olive Oil + Rx: Research continues to show that olive oil may help prevent cancers because of its polyphenols. The American Cancer Society stands by its five to nine servings of vegetables and fruits per day, which may also lower your risk of developing cancer, which increases with age. And, of course, olive oil can help add flavor to fresh produce.

Heart Disease

The Aging Factor: Medical doctors will tell you that the older you get, the more your risks of high cholesterol and high blood pressure go up.

It's Personal: My mother had high blood pressure. I remember that in her thirties, she even had a cardiologist. But, it was her unhealthy lifestyle (smoking, drinking, and stress) that certainly fueled her heart problems. While I have never smoked or had a drop of alcohol, I did inherit her type-A personality, which is linked to heart disease.

Olive Oil + Rx: Research shows that olive oil can help lower the risk of developing heart disease. But, it is the Mediterranean diet and lifestyle (including regular exercise) that can help stave off heart problems. So, remember that fish, whole grains, fruits, vegetables, and getting physical every day along with consuming olive oil may keep you heart-healthy for years. And, learning how to chill is part of the anti–heart disease plan.

Obesity

The Aging Factor: Middle-age spread affects both women and men, thanks to changing hormones and a slower metabolism. Often, body fat ends up on the belly, and this can create health woes from heart disease to diabetes.

It's Personal: As a former hippie, I recall how it was stylish to be thin like models. In my teens, I struggled with bulimia and anorexia. We didn't have names for these eating disorders then, nor were there support groups. I ended up going back to college, and once I had a new life, I learned that healthful food was my friend and overeating or not eating was my enemy.

Olive Oil + Rx: Anecdotal evidence shows that olive oil can suppress the appetite. The older you get, the more you want to stay physically active, to burn off your calories instead of storing body fat. Teaming olive oil with fat-burning foods such as vegetables, whole grains, and fish may also help you keep satisfied, as well as maintain a lean body throughout your life span.

Osteoporosis

The Aging Factor: The "brittle bone" disease can strike at any age. Osteoporosis, the loss of bone density, is often thought of as an older person's disease—but it can strike as early as the thirties, forties, and fifties. But note, the chances of bone loss increase as you age, because your bones become less dense and weaker.

It's Personal: Years ago, I had a neighbor, Ruth, 69, who was a retired widow. I used to watch her walk to the grocery store. It was a sight to see because she had become disfigured with a "dowager's hump." Think of the wicked witch in the *Wizard of Oz*. This image is frightening to many people, like me, who are at risk. As we age, estrogen plummets, especially after menopause, and the incidence of bone loss rises. Women are about four times more apt to develop bone loss. Caucasian (like me) and Asian women are more likely to develop bone loss. Small-boned people—again, women (like me)—are at greater risk.

Olive Oil + Rx: Olive oil solo may help beat bone loss. However, other fatty acids—the "good" fats—also play various roles in bone structure, function, and development. The fact is, fats are necessary for good calcium metabolism and are essential components of cartilage and bone. Best sources: olive oil, fish oil, and flaxseed oil.

Teeth

The Aging Factor: Baby boomers and seniors these days can and do have their own teeth. Dentures are the last resort. In the twenty-first century, we have modern dentistry, from crowns to dental implants, that help us preserve our own smile, unlike our parents in the twentieth century.

It's Personal: Since I was a teenager, I have been on a healthy teeth campaign. I wore braces. I endured cavities and fillings. In my twenties, I had a crown, and then one day, a root canal. Today, while I still have my own teeth—like the majority of boomers and seniors who practice good dental hygiene—I know that I have to floss and brush daily, see the dentist twice a year and use one of those sonic toothbrushes to keep gingivitis and periodontal disease at bay.

Olive Oil + Rx: Perhaps using a water-and-olive-oil rinse to protect your teeth if you grind at night will help keep your pearly whites in good condition. But a healthful diet, such as the Mediterranean eating plan (with minimal sweets), and drinking six to eight 8-ounce glasses of water daily are also musts to keep your teeth forever young.

Vision

The Aging Factor: Glaucoma and macular degeneration are age-related problems. Both can lead to blindness. Plus, with an increased longevity and decreased good nutrition, good eyesight may not be in the cards.

It's Personal: Eyesight is a precious thing that we take for granted until we reach our forties. Then, before we know it, we need reading glasses for the small print in newspapers and on food labels. Later, the glasses are must-haves for the computer. Also, macular degeneration is a frightening eye problem that I have witnessed in two friends. Both are legally blind.

Olive Oil + Rx: Magnesium-rich foods can help prevent glaucoma and improve blood circulation, according to ophthalmologist Robert Abel Jr., M.D., of Wilmington, Delaware. Antioxidant-rich foods (which taste better with olive oil) and vitamin E–rich oils like soybean oil, corn oil, peanut oil, safflower oil, and sesame oil can help protect against macular degeneration, notes Charles Kroll, an optometrist in Chicago, Illinois. These foods can taste better with olive oil—which also contains antioxidant vitamin E.

As I communicate with other aging boomers and seniors, I realize that aging is not fun. I have lost friends and family to both the scourge of heart disease and cancer. However, if we can help ourselves age gracefully and maintain our health, I feel that while it is a challenge, it doesn't have to be the end of our world as we know it.

Spinach and Tomato Quiche with Garlic Oil

❖ ❖ ❖

As a kid, when my mom returned from Europe, she morphed into an experimental chef. I was a down-to-earth picky eater (not much different than now) and would protest any of her spinach dishes. She concocted one recipe ("Pat Special") with ground beef, eggs, spinach, and other no-name ingredients. Other sixties' dishes, like "tamale pie," were also on my plate. The mush consisted of cornmeal, more hamburger, tomatoes, sweet pepper, onion, and fat. One night I rebelled. I refused to eat the cornmeal mush. Upset by my finicky palate, my mother gave in. I feasted on fish sticks and Tater Tots—processed food of the fifties.

As time passed, my taste for food changed—and I am a semi-vegetarian. I'm like Meg Ryan's Sally character in *When Harry Met Sally*. I'm high maintenance, especially when it comes to food, and prefer my quiche to be prepared with the ingredients I want in it. Quiche is a rich custard pie infused with cheese and vegetables (no need for meat). It may have French roots, but it's also a favorite dish to eat for brunch or dinner here in America. I give this grown-up quiche recipe of mine a Mediterranean spin. My mother would be proud. And yes, I've finally acquired a taste for fresh spinach.

2 tablespoons garlic olive oil

1 tablespoon European-style butter

¼ cup red onion, diced

¼ cup organic fresh baby spinach, thinly sliced

1¼ cups mix of green and red bell pepper and zucchini, chopped

1 teaspoon Herbes de
    Provence (a blend of
    basil, fennel seed, marjo-
    ram, rosemary, sage,
    thyme, and lavender)
    (save ½ cup for topping)
4 organic brown eggs,
    beaten
1 cup organic half-and-half

1 tablespoon light olive oil
1 (9-inch) store-bought re-
    frigerated pie crust*
1 cup low-fat mozzarella,
    shredded
2 slices mozzarella,
    chopped
12 cherry tomatoes, sliced
    in half

In a skillet, melt garlic olive oil and butter. Stir-fry red onion and vegetables and herbs. Set aside. In a mixing bowl, beat eggs; add half-and-half. Brush olive oil on uncooked pie crust. Top with half of veggie mixture. Sprinkle with half of cheese. Repeat. Pour milk-egg mixture on top. Spread spinach; place tomato halves on top. Bake at 400° for about 45 minutes or till golden brown and firm. Makes 8–10 servings.

*If you want a heart-healthy pie crust, turn to the Olive Oil Crust in this book and do it yourself. Or find a store-bought crust with no trans fat.

In Part 5, "Olive Oil Home Remedies," you'll discover some amazing ways to use olive oil to help you feel better and look great—whether it's for moisturizing your skin from head to toe or keeping your companion animals forever younger, too.

THE GOLDEN SECRETS TO REMEMBER

✓ You can take years off your biological age by changing your diet and lifestyle—and olive oil can play a part.

✓ As health insurance rates go up, if you increase the "good" fats and lose the "bad" fats, you can lower your risk of developing age-related diseases.

✓ Teaming antioxidant-rich red wine and balsamic vinegars with Mediterranean diet foods that are rich in resveratrol may help you lose body fat as well as win the aging game.

✓ Omega-3 oils can help stave off the aches and pains of arthritis as you age.

✓ Polyphenol-rich olive oil may help to lower your risk of developing age-related cancers.

✓ Heart-healthy olive oil can help you maintain healthy blood pressure, cholesterol, and blood sugar numbers, which will beat heart disease and diabetes.

✓ Research proves olive oil can help you maintain your weight (a problem in aging boomers and seniors) by keeping hunger pangs at bay.

✓ "Good" fats such as olive oil and other fatty acids strengthen bone density, which can help you beat bone loss (at any age).

✓ Olive oil as a protective mouth rinse, as well as a healthful diet and regular dental checkups, can preserve your pearly whites.

PART 5

OLIVE OIL HOME REMEDIES

1 3

Cures from Your Kitchen

> *Only the sea itself seems as ancient a part of the*
> *region as the olive and its oil, that like no other*
> *products of nature, have shaped civilizations*
> *from remotest antiquity to the present.*
> —Lawrence Durrell[1]

On June 26, 2007, I like hundreds of people in South Lake Tahoe, endured enormous stress due to an out of control wildfire. Stress is triggered partly by the sensitivity of our sympathetic system, which jump-starts the fight-or-flight reaction. So when the pressure is on, up go our pulse rate, respiration and muscle tension. The bottom line: I was scared and my companion animals were excited.

Once I realized the fire was too close to home, I chose to flee to escape the smoke inhalation, helicopters, sirens, ash, automated evacuation telephone calls, gridlock due to closed roads, and mass chaos of the Angora Fire.

I grabbed my must-have essentials: two dogs, one cat, a brother (in denial), a pile of clothes, a laptop computer, pet food and supplies, and my purse full of personal items. Once we settled in at a pet-friendly hotel in Reno, Nevada, I realized hour by hour that I didn't have two items I'm used to having for comfort, beauty, and pesky human and pet ailments.

I didn't have extra virgin olive oil (which I use on my skin, feet, hands and hair) nor did I have vinegar for Simon, my dog's sore nose (evidently his was bit by something) and his abraded paws due to the hot asphalt and wet grass during his walks). It hit me. I missed having both oil and vinegar—two universal liquids—for emergencies, like this unforgettable one, because they have so many uses when you are away and back at home.

Chances are, olive oil, coconut oil, and other oils—your everyday household products—contain even more extraordinary healing powers that you might not know about. The next time you need a natural remedy for an ailment, check this list first to see if a cure is as close as your kitchen cabinet or pantry.

I'll describe common health ailments and cosmetic problems, from A to Z, and provide at-home healing-oil folk remedies. Some treatments can be used inside and others outside the body. Keep in mind these are based on anecdotal evidence. There are no hard-hitting studies to back up their effectiveness and make it conclusive.

30 Amazing Oil Remedies

Did you know that olive oil (and other oils) is considered one of the most popular folk remedies? Well, if this surprises you, read on, and you'll see why oil remedies are good to have in your home, wherever you live. But note, use common sense, and consult your doctor, before starting any new treatments—folk remedies or not.

1 BEAT BLADDER INFECTIONS Bladder infection coming on? You begin to urinate but feel a burning pain. It may be a bladder infection, also called a urinary tract infection (UTI). Worse, you may feel an urgency to urinate and pain in the lower back and pelvic area. Bacteria can cause bladder infections. Also, the hormonal changes that hit at menopause can trigger UTIs. Some medical experts believe that when estrogen declines, the pH level of the vagina changes and the number of good bacteria declines.

What Oil Remedy to Use: One teaspoon of olive oil and one teaspoon of garlic juice mixed in a glass of warm water. Drink three times a day, preferably before meals. It also may be helpful to drink cranberry juice as a preventative measure.

Why You'll Like It: It's a pain to take time out to go to the doctor. It's also a pain to deal with the side effects that come with the antibiotics commonly used to treat bladder infections.

2 BABY SKIN BURNS Ever accidentally burn yourself while cooking, stoking wood in a fireplace, or drinking a beverage that is just too hot? Like bladder infections, burns can be painful, and the pain can last for a while. Since biblical times, people have turned to the almighty olive and its oil to help heal burns naturally.

What Oil Remedy to Use: Apply extra virgin olive oil on your burn three or four times daily.

Why You'll Like It: Not only is it natural, but olive oil doesn't have a strong medicine smell. Also, its antibiotic effect does the job. If you burn your mouth or lip, olive oil is gentle and edible.

3 BYE-BYE BRUXISM In the twenty-first century, people are preserving their pearly whites throughout their lifetime, unlike in the twentieth century, when dentures were more common. These days, if you brush your teeth and floss regularly, get checkups twice a year, and have dental cleanings as needed, you have a good chance of keeping your smile. And, olive oil may help, too.

"Olive oil has been shown to decrease tooth wear, but only in small studies where it was used to minimize the damage caused by grinding (bruxism). It acted as a lubricant in combination with an acrylic tooth guard," notes California olive oil expert John Deane, M.D.

What Oil Remedy to Use: Before bedtime, rinse your mouth with an emulsion of olive oil and water to decrease plaque (the sticky substance that can create inflammation of the gums or gingivitis).

Why You'll Like It: What's not to like? If this easy, all-natural mouth rinse can help to preserve your teeth, why not give it a go? Plus, some mouthwash rinses are strong and can discolor your teeth temporarily, until you have them professionally cleaned by a dental hygienist.

4 CURE A COUGH Do you have a nagging cough? A tickle in your throat can be more annoying than a skin burn. Often, coughs occur after a cold or are linked to an allergy. The fact is, if you're hacking during the day or night, you (and others around you) have one sentence on the brain: "How can I make that annoying cough go away?"

What Oil Remedy to Use: Take 1 tablespoon of olive oil as needed.

Why You'll Like It: It may be just what you need to help you chase away that cough because it will lubricate a tickle in your throat. A bonus: Olive oil doesn't contain undesirable ingredients (for example, codeine) that commercial syrups do, and it may even taste better than some.

5 CAN CONSTIPATION Speaking of annoyances . . . Feeling irregular? You're hardly alone. Often, a change in climate or travel can wreak havoc on your regularity. Constipation can affect you (at any age). Forget cod liver oil. It doesn't taste very good, and there is a more practical remedy.

What Oil Remedy to Use: Take 1 tablespoon of extra virgin olive oil with vegetables and fruits. Don't forget to enjoy five to nine servings daily.

Why You'll Like It: Olive oil and veggies is an all-natural remedy that works. Increasing your intake of fresh produce, drinking plenty of water—six to eight 8 ounce glasses daily—and getting regular exercise also can help you stay regular.

6 CODDLE CUTICLES Dry cuticles? Many people (at any age), especially those who live in cold climates, suffer from bouts of dry hands and dry cuticles. Worse, if you tear the hanging skin, it can lead to an open cut or wound. If you ignore dry cuticles, you can end up with an infection.

What Oil Remedy to Use: Try applying olive oil directly to your hands and cuticles twice daily. Also, use an olive oil–based soap.

Why You'll Like It: Teaming the two home cures works like a charm. One devout user told me, "I keep a small container of it handy for rubbing into my cuticles. Keeps them super soft and smelling less artificial than most moisturizers on the market these days."

7 EASE AN EARACHE Ears throb? Like a cough or irregular bowel habits, an earache can drive you crazy. I endured an ear infection (due to the cold, dry winter weather). So, I went to the bathroom cabinet to reach for those prescribed eardrops. The date had expired. This time around, it was in the fall, and I knew it was swimmer's ear due to a regular routine of swimming laps at the gym. It was late at night, so I turned to olive oil instead.

What Oil Remedy to Use: Put a few drops of olive oil in the ear canal. Repeat as needed.

Why You'll Like It: For one, if it's a minor earache, olive oil, which is believed to have mild antibiotic properties, can and does get rid of the ache and heal the pain.

8 DUMP DANDRUFF Dry flakes and dry scalp? It can be a pesky cosmetic issue (unlike an ear infection), since dandruff can get out of control. Before you run to the dermatologist, consider using both conditioning olive oil and antibacterial vinegar, which kill the bacteria that is believed to be the cause.

What Oil Remedy to Use: Beauty experts suggest combining both vinegar and olive oil with water. I suggest 2 tablespoons of apple cider vinegar, 2 tablespoons of spring water, and 2 tablespoons of extra virgin olive oil. Mix them together, then massage them into your scalp. Rinse after 20 minutes, and shampoo.

Why You'll Like It: Ever smell dandruff shampoos? Ugh! The unnatural scent and harsh chemicals are enough to make you scream out loud in disgust before handling the toxic-smelling shampoo, let alone putting it on your sacred crown. Opt for a natural oil remedy, and see if it works for you.

9 DISS DIAPER RASH Almost everyone has seen a diaper rash, which is an infant's reddened bottom. There are store-bought remedies, but if you aren't near a store, what to do? Many olive oil experts say olive oil has been used to treat diaper rash in olive-producing countries such as Italy. Antonio gives kudos to his grandmother for her "washed oil" special remedy, which works for both a sunburn and a "baby's inflamed bottom."

What Oil Remedy to Use: Use 2 teaspoons of extra virgin olive oil with 1 teaspoon of water. Shake these two ingredients until you get a pasty emulsion, a sort of cream ready to be spread on your body.

Why You'll Like It: Not only does Antonio validate this remedy, but as a "mom" with three fur children, I can tell you that if there is a natural remedy for an ailment, I will turn to it before using a product with chemicals in it. So, Antonio's grandma's "magic ointment" may make both you and your child or grandchild tickled pink when it clears up the redness on baby.

10 FIX YOUR SORE FEET All of us have had to stand on our feet longer than we would have liked, whether it was to feed a baby with a diaper rash, to wait in line with a baby at the grocery store or airport, or perhaps to take a hike solo for fun. If you have been there, done that, you may have wished for a quick cure to soothe away the pain. Some olive oil fans who believe in its folklore magic also believe it can pamper tired feet.

What Oil Remedy to Use: Try a soak in a pan of warm water. Dilute 3 drops of lavender essential oil, 2 drops of eucalyptus essential oil, and 2 drops of lemon essential oil in 2 teaspoons of olive oil. Add to a footbath.

Why You'll Like It: A relaxing soak can ease the cares of the day, and the olive oil combination relieves foot soreness.

11 FORGET FIBROMYALGIA Want to shake aches and pains in your muscles? If you have tenderness in eleven or more of the eighteen "tender points," which include the back of the neck, lower back, and lateral hips, you may have fibromyalgia. Or, if your tender points don't reach eleven you still may have a flare-up, especially during stressful times, or when cold-weather changes hit.

What Oil Remedy to Use: Eating an antioxidant-rich diet complete with vegetables, fruits, and fish drizzled with olive oil, which has anti-inflammatory properties, may help. Also, try massaging the areas on your body that ache.

Why You'll Like It: If you can get relief from sore, stiff muscles, you will feel more comfortable and will be able to resume normal daily activities.

12 GOOD-BYE GALLBLADDER PROBLEMS It's no secret that obesity is a risk factor for gallstones. Also, if you have cholesterol woes and eat fatty foods, you may be experiencing gallbladder trouble. Your first line of action should be to up your fiber intake, eat a low-fat diet, and lose some unwanted weight. Some natural-cure practitioners tout an olive oil remedy to cleanse excess refined carbs, sugar, and fat.

What Oil Remedy to Use: Try approximately 2 tablespoons of olive oil chased by $\frac{1}{2}$ cup grapefruit or lemon juice each morning for one week.

Why You'll Like It: If it works in conjunction with your new gallbladder diet and lifestyle, you may not be haunted by developing gallstones or needing surgery.

13 GOOD RIDDANCE TO GINGIVITIS Puffy gums? Pink toothbrush? Bleeding gums? Welcome to gingivitis—inflammation of the gums. Certainly, regular brushing, flossing, and dental checkups and cleanings are preventative measures. But can olive oil help fight red and swollen gums and stave off periodontal problems, which can lead to tooth loss?

What Oil Remedy to Use: Rinse your mouth with an emulsion of olive oil and water.

Why You'll Like It: According to Dr. Deane, small studies have shown that this olive oil remedy can decrease plaque, the sticky substance that can form into tartar, which only a dental cleaning can remove. If you want to ward off periodontal disease and save your pearly whites, it may be worth a try.

14 HALT HAIR LOSS Both men and women may need to cope with thinning hair, which can be due to many causes, from hormones or genetics to nutritional deficiencies. If you're not getting enough essential fatty acids or vitamins A and E—all components of olive oil—this home cure may help you maintain the strength of your hair.

What Oil Remedy to Use: Take 1 tablespoon of extra virgin olive oil daily or use it in your food, especially foods with essential fatty acids, such as slivered almonds and tuna.

Why You'll Like It: Olive oil incorporated into your diet can help keep your hair nourished and soft. Vitamin A helps keep hair strong, and vitamin E retards the aging of skin cells. But note, if you are a man, you may consider shaving your head, which to many people is attractive. Using olive oil will give the skin on your head a healthful sheen.

15 HANG UP A HANGOVER Killer headache? Ever suffer the day after from drinking too much alcohol? The symptoms can be nasty, including a bad headache, nausea, and sensitivity to light and sound. Rather than deal, it might be easier to try an olive oil cure.

What Oil Remedy to Use: On the Internet, you can find a variety of references to a "prairie cocktail," which is a concoction of olive oil, tomato ketchup, and vinegar.

Why You'll Like It: Well, one desperate gentleman claimed it made him sick. But it is believed that the olive oil cleanses the gallbladder and liver, as well as soothes the tummy.

16 HIT ILLNESS WITH ANTIBACTERIAL HAND SOAP Want to avoid getting sick during the cold and flu season? Since washing your hands often can help stave off contagious illnesses, which usually make the rounds in the fall and winter, a good antibacterial soap can help you. One holiday season, I forgot to buy hand soap. I had to create a quick remedy. I had purchased antibacterial dish soap, but I thought, "This is going to be too harsh on my hands." So, I turned to versatile olive oil.

What Oil Remedy to Use: Pour 3 parts antibacterial dish soap and 1 part extra virgin olive oil in a handy soap dispenser.

Why You'll Like It: It works double duty. Not only do you clean your hands well each time you wash them, but you get a soothing, all-natural moisturizer, too.

17 HANG UP HOT FLASHES Menopausal woes can and do often include pesky hot flashes or temperature ups and downs before, during, and after menopause, aka "The Change." In Asian countries, hot flashes are not a frequent problem according to research because women consume soy, which may help keep hot flashes at bay.

What Oil Remedy to Use: Take 1 or 2 tablespoons of olive oil, flaxseed oil, or soybean oil per day. Or, drizzle a tablespoon or 2 on five servings of vegetables daily. (Include asparagus, beans, carrots, corn, dried seaweed, garlic, green pepper, onions, squash, and yams.)

Why You'll Like It: By using olive oil with vegetables, you may find yourself at a normal temperature rather than feeling waves of heat or turning red while onlookers stare at you as though you were an alien from another planet.

18 LACKLUSTER LIBIDO Not in the mood? You may have read that olive oil can rev up your sex drive or jump-start your (or your lover's) libido. I haven't found any data to prove that olive oil is the cure-all for a lackluster love life, but I do know there are studies that showed sexual performance was enhanced after taking a variety of nutrients including vitamins A, C, E, and B complex and the minerals selenium and zinc. And remember, olive oil is rich in vitamin E (an antioxidant believed to be a sex vitamin).

What Oil Remedy to Use: Eat a low-fat, nutrient-rich meal and drizzle olive oil over it on a regular basis and before a lovemaking session. Also, some people believe porcini olive oil (fresh wild mushrooms infused in olive oil) may act as an aphrodisiac.

Why You'll Like It: Pairing olive oil with a nutrient-dense diet (or porcini olive oil) may do the trick in the bedroom. A healthful, low-fat diet may help to maintain your blood vessels and blood flow, claim medical doctors. That's important in enhancing healthful orgasms in both men and women.

19 MASSAGE MUSCLE ACHES Ever suffer from a strained muscle due to working out at the gym or doing too much indoor or outdoor housework? Actually, muscle aches and pains can affect you at any age. After swimming laps at a resort pool, bringing in plenty of hardwood for a winter fire, walking the dogs, and vacuuming (whew!), my upper back and inner shoulders throbbed. I called a local personal trainer, and he suggested calling a masseuse. Her fee: $120 per hour. I decided to try a healing oil and my own two hands.

What Oil Remedy to Use: Warm 1 cup of olive oil in the microwave. Apply it as a massage oil. (If you have a significant other, this can be even more delightful. But doing it solo can work, too.)

Why You'll Like It: The warmth of the oil immediately re-laxes stiff muscles, and the massage motion also loosens up tight muscles and tendons. Plus, you can spend that hundred bucks in multiple other ways to pamper yourself, such as to join a gym that has a hot tub, steam room, and sauna—other ways to soothe your aches and pains away.

The Magic of Scents, Massage, and Oil

Did you know that using olive oil combined with essential oils from aromatic plants can help you to relax the body, mind, and spirit? This isn't news. The art of using aromatic essential oils for physical and mental well-being goes back to the Egyptians. Some of the popular oils for good health include chamomile, lavender, lemon, jasmine, peppermint, rosemary, tea tree, and sandalwood.

To use essential oils, like these powerful healers, you'll need to use a "carrier oil," that is, any oil that is used to dilute pure essential oils. Carrier oils help essential oils spread more evenly, and they help conserve the use of costly essential oils. A common dilution is 10 to 15 drops of essential oil to 1 ounce of carrier oil. Carrier oils are extracted from nuts, kernels, seeds, and other parts of plants.

Almond oil and sesame oil are used for massage. Olive oil is used for healing and lubricating the skin, as well as for massage. (See more in Chapter 8.)

According to massage therapists, there are different types of massage. Here are the most common types:

- Stroking—uses long and firm strokes using the hands or thumbs to trace the outer shape of the body.

- Kneading—works on different muscle groups by lifting, rolling, and squeezing them.
- Friction—uses circular strokes on the deeper muscles and tendons. This technique moves against the grain of a muscle.
- Percussion—uses gentle drumming motions, often on the back.
- Vibration—shakes the muscles back and forth.

Callie's Reviving Massage Oil

This activating eucalyptus massage oil is effective for sore and aching muscles. Combine the following essential oils:

    20 drops eucalyptus
    20 drops lavender
    20 drops rosewood
    5 drops chamomile
    5 drops peppermint

Add 36 drops of this blend to 3 ounces olive oil. Shake briefly, and massage a small amount into tired, achy muscles and joints.

20 LOSE LICE It seems like kids pick up these pesky creatures at school. The question is, can olive oil be a lice buster or not? Frankly, the answer is not conclusive. Olive oil can zap lice sometimes, sometimes not. So, the verdict is out whether the olive oil remedy is 100 percent effective.

What Oil Remedy to Use: Apply olive oil to the hair and leave it on at least a half hour, according to folks who claim this home cure can do the job. Then, shampoo twice.

You may have to try a series of olive oil applications to the head. Olive oil applicator bottles can be purchased at www.headliceinfo.com, where you can also find out everything else you ever wanted to know about lice but were afraid to ask.

Why You'll Like It: If this natural suffocating agent does work for you or your child, you'll be happy because olive oil is a much gentler treatment than the harsh commercial products, which contain pesticides.

21 PEEL AWAY PSORIASIS Psoriasis (which can be worse than lice, which is a short-term problem) can range from mild, in which a few small red patches appear on the elbows or feet, to severe, with unsightly, scaly areas covering the entire body. A friend of mine told me that her cousin suffered from psoriasis, and it truly is more than a cosmetic problem for some people, according to the National Psoriasis Foundation.

What Oil Remedy to Use: Before bedtime, apply olive oil generously to the affected area, then massage. Rinse in the morning. Repeat as needed.

Why You'll Like It: One mom, Jackie Larson of Dallas, Texas, attests that olive oil did the trick. "My son had terrible inherited psoriasis in his scalp. A hairdresser saw this and suggested rubbing olive oil deeply into his scalp. I applied it liberally to his scalp, enough to get his hair wet with it, completely removing any dried skin and thoroughly massaging it in," she recalls. Jackie left the oil in overnight and washed it out in the morning. "Within a matter of days, the flaking had stopped and within a few weeks, his scalp was essentially clear. We repeat when necessary," she notes.

Also, steroid creams can cause additional thinning of the

skin. Olive oil is believed to feel better to apply than petro-leum jelly or if it works and you nip psoriasis in the bud you won't have to turn to prescription drugs.

22 SOOTHE A STOMACHACHE Upset tummy? Diarrhea? Some folk remedy fans believe olive oil can put your queasy feelings to rest. Also, Edgar Cayce believed the oil adds to the "elasticity of the functioning of the intestinal tract." It doesn't take a crystal ball for you to sense that the smooth liquid can relax an irritated stomach.

What Oil Remedy to Use: Take 1/4 teaspoon every four hours.

Why You'll Like It: If you are nowhere near a pharmacy or a doctor but you are feeling queasy, you'll love this olive oil cure.

23 STOP SUNBURN Skin woes, whether psoriasis or sunburn, can be a problem that lingers for years. Exposure to the ultraviolet rays of sunlight is the main cause of sunburn. I can personally attest that it can be worse if you live in a high altitude, near water, or in an exotic region such as Hawaii or Mexico. I am fair-skinned and I got bad sunburns (second degree) both in Las Vegas and on the Big Island. Since I certainly don't want to get premature wrinkles or skin cancer, I did wear sunscreen. But sometimes it's just not enough.

What Oil Remedy to Use: According to Firenze, use olive oil to soothe the reddened skin and even the blisters that follow sun exposure.

Why You'll Like It: Well, it won't burn like vinegar does. Plus, the silky texture of olive oil pampers a painful burn without pain or a pesky odor. But it's best to use sunscreen and shun sunbathing for sport.

24 TEND TENDONITIS Shoulder ache? You may have entered painful tendonitis land when your tendons—which connect muscle to bone—become inflamed the way gum tissue often does. I personally can attest to this painful woe, which affected my shoulders after overdoing it with hand weights. Often, it is exercise-related, especially if you do too much. Research shows that olive oil may lessen the aches and pains of bursitis, in which joints become irritated. Both pains are caused by overuse, often from exercise or tasks that require repetitive motions.

What Oil Remedy to Use: Try 1 tablespoon of olive oil before breakfast. If you want to heal faster, try massaging oil into the tender spots as well.

Why You'll Like It: If it works, you will like the fact that you don't have aches and pains from the inflamed regions. Also, it is easier and less time-consuming than icing, which can work in conjunction with this home remedy.

25 TAME TOENAIL FUNGUS Brittle toenails? Since my mid-thirties, I have had dry and brittle toenails. At one time, I was getting professional pedicures twice a month. The pedicurist, from Vietnam, applied an oil on my toes and fingernails before she applied the polish. I assumed it was something pricey she had purchased at a wholesale store. When I asked her about the miracle worker (it made my nails smooth and not brittle-appearing), she giggled and pointed to a container of a common grocery store brand of vegetable oil.

What Oil Remedy to Use: Apply olive oil or canola oil (any type of lubricating oil can be beneficial) around your toes and nails. However, pure extra virgin olive oil is believed to enhance skin and nail health.

Why You'll Like It: Olive oil is all natural, and it provides an immediate cosmetic effect. Also, the prescription drug that is advertised on television doesn't have a high success rate, and the fact that it necessitates regular blood tests to test for liver problems seems like a red flag to me. Like me, you may prefer to use the accessible oil, which does appear to help camouflage dry and brittle nails (perhaps it's the antioxidant vitamin E that does this) and an earthy-colored polish (some brands include nail strengthener) rather than tamper with my vital organs.

26 TACKLE THAT TOOTHACHE Tooth hurt? If one of your teeth—whether a back molar with a filling or a front capped tooth—is throbbing, the pain isn't fun. You may get images of actor Dustin Hoffman in the 1970s film *Marathon Man* and be willing to turn to a popular old remedy—oil of cloves—until you can get to a dentist who wants to help you.

What Oil Remedy to Use: If you don't have oil of cloves on hand, no worry. Blend 2 tablespoons of whole cloves in a blender until a powder forms. Mix with 1 tablespoon of olive oil. Dab on the tooth as needed.

Why You'll Like It: Oil of cloves is a well-known remedy for toothaches. It can provide temporary relief.

27 TAME SAD Ever hear of seasonal affective disorder (SAD), or the "winter blues"? Shorter days, longer nights, and a cold climate, especially without sunshine, can make you feel depressed, lack energy, and pack on the pounds. No,

I'm not going to say olive oil is the cure-all for SAD, but I do believe it can help you become energized again if you team it with other remedies.

What Oil Remedy to Use: Each day, for lunch or dinner or both meals, drizzle olive oil on a dark, leafy green salad with plenty of fresh vegetables. To sleep like a baby, take 1 tablespoon of flaxseed oil before bedtime.

Why You'll Like It: If you eat lots of veggies teamed with olive oil, which can fill you up, you may not fill out. Also, if you get a good night's sleep, you will be less likely to overeat when your energy fizzles throughout the day. Better sleep will make you feel better, and you're more apt to want to exercise, which can help burn calories and fight winter weight gain and depression.

28 TREAT SKIN DAMAGE Toenails often are exposed only in the summertime, but your face is seen daily. During your forties (and earlier if you are fair-skinned), your oil glands become less active, which means moisturizing becomes more important. Although all of the antioxidant skin nutrients are key to younger-looking skin, vitamins A, C, and E—well-touted skin rejuvenators—may play even bigger roles, according to dermatologists and researchers in Melbourne, Australia.

Used topically, olive oil—rich in vitamin E—has benefits such as protecting skin against ultraviolet light and reducing the appearance of fine lines and wrinkles. Used internally, it may even help stall the aging process. Eating foods that contain monounsaturated fats, like olive oil, may prevent skin cell damage. Take a look at ageless beauties like Sophia Loren and Loni Anderson, who have given kudos to olive oil.

What Oil Remedy to Use: Dab olive oil on the areas of the skin and face where wrinkles show, and lightly massage at bedtime. Also, include olive oil, along with other antioxidant-rich foods such as vegetables, fresh fruits, and legumes in your daily menus.

Why You'll Like It: It may work to minimize those laugh lines. Plus, Botox and collagen injections are not cheap and not painless.

29 UNIVERSAL EMERGENCY During Mother Nature's wrath, from tornadoes and hurricanes to snowstorms and earthquakes, it's good to have a cure-all product on hand in case of a power outage. Prepare now by putting together a box of emergency supplies. Make sure to include medications that you, your family, and your pet take, as well as a first-aid kit and handbook.

What Oil Remedy to Use: Purchase a large can of extra virgin olive oil (or two), and store it with your emergency supplies. (Note: Bottles can break during a disaster; plastic can react with oil in time.)

Why You'll Like It: Olive oil has healing powers. Rather than trying to put every type of ailment remedy in your emergency supplies box, it's more practical and cost-effective to have one cure that works for many ailments such as burns, cuts, earaches, and sore muscles.

30 VANQUISH VAGINAL DRYNESS A lackluster sex life for women can be connected to lack of lubrication, which can make lovemaking uncomfortable. Olive oil has been used as a sexual lubricant since historical times, but times change. In the twenty-first century, if you're a woman (or man), you know that lovemaking can sizzle if a woman suffers from vaginal dryness, which can occur because of out-of-whack hormones, not being in the mood, infection, and other physical and psychological reasons. But if you think olive oil is the perfect natural oil-based lubricant, think again.

There are some very important guidelines to consider. For one, oils can damage latex condoms and sex toys. Also, olive oil can often be a woman's worst enemy if she is prone to pesky vaginal infections. Since oil clings, it may be a bacteria magnet.

What Oil Remedy to Use: Olive oil works best as a pre-sex enhancer. That means, use edible oils for a sensual massage, hugging, and cuddling. In addition, olive oil–based foods can be erotic shared in bed. Use olive oil as a sexual lubricant *only* with polyurethane female and male condoms, according to Birth Control–Planned Parenthood of Golden Gate. For self-pleasuring, some men have no complaints about olive oil doing the job.

Why You'll Like It: Use caution when applying olive oil directly to your or your mate's private parts. Before you flaunt olive oil behind closed doors, consult your physician. If you get a thumbs-up, enjoy an all-natural sexual enhancer—both sensual and scentless.

UNUSUAL CURES WITH HEALING OILS

Did you know olive oil isn't the only healing oil that provides home cures that can work for you? There are so many different cooking oils with amazing do-it-yourself cures. Sure, some of these remedies are folklore; others like coconut oil (touted by celebs that use it for a variety of its health perks) come with anecdotal evidence; and some, such as canola oil, are backed up by a stamp of approval from medical researchers.

After I wrote the first edition of *The Healing Powers of Olive Oil*, I used extra virgin olive oil for home cures, including an earache, cracked skin, a spider bite, and wasp sting—all culprits that paid me a visit while I enjoyed the mountain lifestyle. These days, my kitchen pantry is stocked with other oils, too, including coconut oil and macadamia nut oil, that can and do the job.

Personally, I prefer to use a variety of these oils inside and outside my body, as my first line of defense for certain conditions, such as skin and hair issues during the dry wintertime. But that doesn't mean I ignore using healing oils, such as sesame oil and flaxseed oil, by not incorporating them into my diet.

Pairing healing oils inside the body and outside the body is the best way to get the best results from head to toe. So take a look at some of these healing oils, including almond oil, coconut oil, flaxseed oil, hempseed oil, macadamia nut oil, red palm oil, sesame oil, and canola oil, which can be used in cooking but also as home cures. Do consult with your health care practitioner before using any new healing oil for an ailment. (And don't forget, olive oil can also be used for most if not all of these home remedies, too.)

AGE SPOTS (Preventing brown blotches with coconut oil) Brown frecklelike circles on your face, hands, arms, and legs seem to appear on both men and women when Old Man Time pays a visit. Some people may be more prone to getting these spots due to sun exposure or genes. The way I see it, we can go with the flow and embrace our spots like wrinkles and gray hair—or fight it with cosmestic surgery or naturally.

What Oil Remedy to Use: Rub a bit of coconut oil onto age spots, whether they are on your face or hands. Do this three times per day.

Why You'll Like It: No promises that all of your age spots will be gone forever and your skin will look like it did in your twenties; however, the odds are good that your spots may appear lighter and your skin smoother, and that in itself may make the spots seem less noticeable. Proponents of coconut oil believe the anti-age spot potential is due to antioxidants perks. Evidently, these good guys may win the battle of oxidation (think of an apple cut and let out in the air and how it browns due to exposure to light).

ATHLETE'S FOOT (Zapping inflamed feet by using the right oil and vinegar) Age spots, like aging, has its woes, but athlete's foot can occur at any age and is pesky too. This ailment is often picked up in gym locker rooms if you go barefoot, since you are exposed to the environment where bugs are found. This, in turn, can result in red feet, especially in between the toes.

What Oil Remedy to Use: Mix 1 tablespoon coconut oil with 1 tablespoon apple cider vinegar. Use this mixture twice a day.

Why You'll Like It: There's many reasons why you may find this treatment to your liking. It's natural, it's inexpensive, and it doesn't smell as some over-the-counter remedies. This home cure contains lauric acid, an ingredient that makes it an antiviral and antibacterial worker, much like vinegar. You have the anti-fungal properties in vinegar paired with the anti-inflammatory effects of the coconut oil. So if you let the oil and vinegar team do its job, you may just beat a bout of athlete's foot.

BACK PAIN (Curbing aches with oils) Itchy feet are annoying, but an aching back is miserable and doesn't discriminate with gender or age. Personally, I endured a bout of sciatica in my middle years due to a sore back from shoveling snow. Often, the back can hurt when we overdo work or play. Worse, muscles can tense up, and the pain worsens, and it is a challenge to put it out of mind. A heating pad and hot tub or massage can help loosen tight muscles—that's where healing oils come into play.

What Oil Remedy to Use: Try using a generous amount of warm oil, including an almond or a sesame oil massage base with other healing oils, such as coconut oil or olive oil. You can do your upper back and lower back without a partner or professional masseuse. Try twice a day. Shower after.

Why You'll Like It: A good massage with a healing oil will relax your mind and body. The aroma of almond oil is soothing and can help you chill, making aches lessen. It's healthier than taking medication, and it is inexpensive.

BLOAT (Beating water weight with the best oil) Back pain is a pain, but feeling and looking bloated isn't just a cosmetic woe. Years ago, I wrote an article on fat-burning foods. Popcorn was one of the 14 edibles. It's high in fiber, low-fat, low-cal, and no trans fat, especially if you lose the fake butter and salt. It's a super-stress-relieving food because of the crunch, and it can help you get rid of extra water weight, too.

What Oil Remedy to Use: Drizzle 1 or 2 tablespoons of warmed-up red palm oil on top of 2 cups of air-popped popcorn.

Why You'll Like It: Pairing red palm oil with nutritious popcorn is going to give you a double punch of nutrients. This oil contains antioxidant vitamins A and E. Plus, it has a buttery flavor that'll titillate your taste buds and, combined with fiber-rich popcorn, will fill you up not out. As a popcorn lover, I did give this healing oil recipe a go and discovered it was different, and gave it an exotic flair.

BODY FAT (Fighting pudge by enjoying fatty oils) Did you know extra weight and body fat can trigger back pain? It can. And adding good fat to your diet can help you lose unwanted fat and lower your body mass index. Move over, olive oil, because avocado oil and macadamia oil can help you burn fat. These oils boost your energy. Also, they trigger the release of CCK (cholecystokinin)—a hormone that signals to your brain that you're full and should stop eating.

What Oil Remedy to Use: Opt for avocado oil or macadamia oil in a salad full of fat-burning seasonal vegetables.

Why You'll Like It: These two oils taste different than olive oil, so you'll get a nice change, as well as monounsaturated fats, which will give you the feeling of satisfaction after a small meal.

CANKER/COLD SORES (Ending sores faster with the right oil) Backaches to body fat can wreak havoc on your overall health, while canker sores or small ulcers in the mouth can cause big pain for days and make a backache seem like a walk in the park (well sort of). If you've ever fallen victim to one of these mean-spirited sores, it's likely you'd be willing to try anything to get rid of the ache.

What Oil Remedy to Use: Rinse with warm salt water. Then, with a cotton swab, dab a bit of coconut oil (from a capsule or jar) or extra virgin olive oil on the canker sore. Repeat three times a day.

Why You'll Like It: It's soothing like any oil. But because it's thicker, it adheres to your skin better and offers a coating. If you can keep your tongue off the ulcer (this is a task!), it will heal faster. Coconut oil contains anti-inflammatory and antibacterial properties. Also, unlike bad-tasting over-the-counter remedies, coconut oil tastes good.

CRACKED FEET (Creating smooth feet with a natural oil) You may think canker sores are painful, but if you ever fall victim to alligator skin–like rough, red, weathered feet with crevices, you might rather deal with the mouth malady. Cracked feet are an unsightly cosmetic problem, but crevices can turn into health issues, too. Inflammation can lead to pain when walking, wearing shoes, and can even lead to an infection. This, in turn, means a small problem like cracked feet end up being a big problem. Dry skin on the soles of your feet are more common in colder months where there is a lack of humidity.

What Oil Remedy to Use: Try using two coconut capsules topically once a day, preferably before bedtime. Break open each capsule and rub the creamy oil generously on the bottoms of both feet. Cover with 100 percent cotton socks. Repeat daily.

Why You'll Like It: Coconut oil is known for its anti-inflammatory and antibacterial properties. It can help hydrate and soothe painful skin irritations, including cracked feet. Not only does it work, but the texture and aroma of this oil is a pleasant surprise and a miracle worker.

DRY SCALP (Taming flakes by using oils) There's a link between skin and hair. You are what you eat, and you represent the health and beauty of your hair. Many of the same nutrients that protect your hair also nourish your hair. Eating nutrient-dense foods is necessary for your hair follicles to regenerate to keep your hair in its growth phase.

A lack of protein can result in thin, dry hair. So including more protein-packed foods like lean poultry, fish, and yogurt, can help healthy up your crowning glory. Also, essential fatty acids found in canola oil teamed with protein can be a hair helper.

What Oil Remedy to Use: For internal use, use canola oil or coconut oil and a source of protein every day in your diet. Five to six teaspoons is the recommended amount. Plus, topically use macadamia nut oil by putting a small amount onto your hands and directly on your hair after it's washed and dried naturally.

Why You'll Like It: The natural nut oil instantly makes your hair feel like silk. It helps stave off frizzy hair year-round and provides a bit of a shine.

FATIGUE (Ending lack of energy by consuming oil-rich foods) Enjoying a healthy crowning glory is nice, but feeling tired is not nice no matter how thick and shiny your locks may be. Sweet coconut oil can help give you a pick-me-up.

It's a healthy saturated fat—touted to be a natural source of medium-chain triglycerides—which are gobbled up by your body to give it a boost of energy.

What Oil Remedy to Use: Add one or two teaspoons in a cold, fresh, seasonal fruit smoothie.

Why You'll Like It: If you're trying to lose weight, coconut oil can help energize you and provide a feeling of fullness. This, in turn, means if you use it in a smoothie, stir-fry, or even a small baked muffin (see recipes section), you will get physical, burn off calories and fat, and not feel deprived.

GINGIVITIS (Preventing inflamed gums with the anti-inflammatory oil) Fatigue can cause your immune system to weaken and sometimes affect your gums to have an inflammation or gingivitis. Welcome to plaque, the film of bacteria. Plaque is food particles and mucus that work together between your teeth and under your gumline. Good dental hygiene can keep your gums healthy, but sometimes it's difficult to keep inflamed gums at bay. Plaque can irritate your gums to become red, swollen, and throbbing. So what can you do besides brush and floss?

What Oil Remedy to Use: Rub a bit of coconut oil from a jar or a capsule on top of the inflamed gum. Repeat as needed. See your dentist for a follow-up visit to provide peace of mind and make sure there isn't an underlying problem.

Why You'll Like It: Over-the-counter medications to ease dental or gum pain contain a lot of ingredients and don't titillate the taste buds. Coconut oil contains anti-inflammatory and antibacterial properties, and the flavor is sweet.

HEMORRHOIDS (Taming a pain in the butt with oils) Inflamed gums are one irritating woe in life, while hemorrhoids are another. Enter irritating rectum piles that look like little balls either external or internal. Theories include that hemorrhoids are swelling veins or blood-filled cushions. Whatever theory is correct, they can affect both men and women—more if you're pregnant, sedentary, strain when going to the bathroom, or aging. It's usually not a serious problem, but it warrants some action. Eating fiber-rich foods and drinking six to eight eight-ounce glasses of water daily can help you become regular, as can regular exercise. But that's not all.

What Oil Remedy to Use: It's been noted in folk medicine that taking a tablespoon of flaxseed oil (or coconut oil or olive oil) each morning in a smoothie is a good dose.

Why You'll Like It: While hemorrhoids aren't life-threatening, they can be a pesky problem that you'll want to take a permanent vacation from. There are over-the-counter topical treatments to help soothe the irritation, but anti-inflammatory coconut oil and olive oil may reduce both the pain, itching, and swelling. It's worth a try to go natural with healing oils like these, and if it doesn't do the trick, consult your health care practitioner.

INSECT BITES (Lessening inflammation with the right oil) If you experience hemorrhoids, an insect bite may seem like a walk in the park amid mosquitoes, which can be painful, too. Two winters ago, I put on my snow garb: jeans, flannel shirt, down vest, ski hat, mittens, neck scarf, and Sorels. Then I went out to the stack of wood buried in the snow by the fence, and for about an hour, I brought it inside the cabin and on a bench closer to the door.

Yes, I complained.

"What am I doing? I'm too old to be doing this. I'm moving to a warm coastal town. Or maybe I'll just run away and book a one-way ticket to the Big Island."

But the cold wasn't my only challenge. After I made a big fire (it took me several years to master this feat) and sat down on my warm waterbed to chill with my fur kids, I logged on to my laptop computer. As I was typing, I felt a tickle and then prick on my cheek. A big brown spider greeted me on the keyboard. It was like a scene out of the film *Arachnophobia*. One tetanus shot later and a swollen cheek and arm, I turned to coconut oil to heal my wounds. It made me feel better (perhaps it was the exotic scent that helped me visualize an exotic oasis without insects) and got me through the pain of the spooky spider adventure in the wintertime.

What Oil Remedy to Use: Try rubbing a small amount of coconut oil on the bite. Repeat as necessary.

Why You'll Like It: Coconut oil has anti-inflammatory properties that may provide a soothing effect to calm the burning and itching of redness on the skin. If it does its job and takes the sting out of the pain, you will be happy. Don't forget the aroma is more pleasant than over-the-counter products that contain a medicinal smell. While the spider was later identified as a brown recluse (toxic but not deadly), I was lucky. If it ever happens again, I will try coconut oil.

INSOMNIA (Getting shut-eye by including oil in your diet) Bites will heal, but if you don't get adequate sleep, your well-being will suffer and be worse than a bug bite.

Sleep restores and replenishes your body and mind. Lack of sleep depletes energy and frazzles nerves. And lack of adequate *zzzs* may compromise your immune system and lower your resistance to illness. While I often can fall asleep within five minutes to the purr of a cat, I am human and have fallen victim to the cycles of sleeplessness. Some doctors believe PMS and menopause (yes, I'm a survivor of both female culprits) might cause shifts in hormonal balances and trigger a bout of insomnia. For moderate insomnia, healing oils combined with good bedtime habits can be a godsend if you don't want to watch infomercials all night long.

What Oil Remedy to Use: Try a light dinner with a stir-fry, or ice cream with sesame oil and lavender olive oil.

Why You'll Like It: Lavender relaxes the nervous system. It's calming and relaxing. Sesame oil is high in omega-6s. It's a natural sedative used in food. If you are lucky enough to have a partner willing to give you a massage, lavender oil and sesame oil can penetrate the skin and help relax you, too.

IRREGULARITY (Taming constipation with oil) Sleep deprivation is a challenge and can make you feel cranky and not your best, much like suffering from not being able to go on a regular basis. Constipation affects everyone sooner or later. It can strike due to many reasons, including lack of fiber in the diet, not drinking enough water, lack of exercise, stress, and even a change in weather or your schedule.

What Oil Remedy to Use: Take 1 tablespoon flaxseed oil in a smoothie once a day. Repeat as needed.

Why You'll Like It: Flaxseed oil boasts soluble fiber. Once you're regular again, you'll like this home cure because it works and is natural.

PERIMENOPAUSE (Stopping symptoms with flaxseed oil) Sleepless nights are one thing, but pair them with hot flashes and you enter the land of "pre-menopaws." Yes, it's true, premenopausal symptoms are sometimes a woman's worst friend. It can feel like premenstrual crankies, cramps, and cravings 30 days a month. Estrogen therapy is frowned upon but living with discomfort during "the change" doesn't make women smile. So what to do? It's time to turn to a natural healing oil for help to ease the pain of physical woes.

What Oil Remedy to Use: Try 1 tablespoon flaxseed oil in smoothies, on cereal, or on a salad.

Why You'll Like It: It's believed by health gurus that the lignans in flaxseed oil are phytoestrogens (estrogenic compounds found in plants). These, in turn, may alleviate pesky menopausal symptoms. Some health professionals have told me this high-lignan component relieves depression, fatigue, and allergies, but the lignans are estrogenlike substances that have balancing effects on serotonin and other mood regulators.

VAGINAL SPERM-FRIENDLY LUBRICATION (Preventing dryness with the right oil) Premenopause does have a mixed bag of physical discomforts as does lack of lubrication during childbearing years. Vaginal dryness can happen to younger women (it's not just an older ladies' dilemma) due to a host of reasons, from not being in the mood to make love, to hormones. Welcome to an all-natural lubricant that won't chase away good sperm.

What Oil Remedy to Use: A sperm-friendly, small amount of canola oil applied topically inside a woman's private parts is all that's needed to help lubricate dry tissue so lovemaking can be more comfortable.

Why You'll Like It: If getting pregnant is your goal but lubrication is needed to boost the mood, using a plant-based oil is best because it won't kill off sperm the way certain over-the-counter lubricants with spermicides can do.

WORRY (Stopping anxiety with stress-reducing oil) Lovemaking can be challenging, but worrying can wreak havoc on our mind, body, and spirit. The following stressors can cause high anxiety and perpetuate worry: death of a spouse or family member, divorce, loss of a job, loss of financial security, personal injury or illness, a new marriage, trouble with a boss or coworkers, and loss of a home. While most "what-ifs" do not happen—we don't have control over certain situations. Rather than worry about the future, it is better to chill and live life in the present.

What Oil Remedy to Use: Put almond oil to work in a simple massage recipe. Combine 1 ounce almond oil, 3 drops rose oil, and 3 drops lavender oil. Make a base by combining the almond oil and essential oils, and blend. Massage your neck, arms, legs, and feet.

Why You'll Like It: While this calming anti-worry massage oil can be enjoyed with a partner massaging you, you can also do it solo. Touch is a part of soothing your spirit and soul. It can help you relax. Almond oil with its calming scent can help you put your worries to rest, especially with stress-relieving lavender. Candlelight, music, and an almond oil massage is the key to send your worries on a vacation—exhale.

YEAST INFECTION (Stopping inflammation with coconut oil) Worrying happens for all sorts of reasons, and believe it or not, women who take a course of antibiotics may be concerned that a vaginal yeast infection complete with inflammation and itching may follow. Welcome to yeast, a common kind of fungus, called *Candida albicans,* which lives in the vagina in normal amounts. If it overgrows, it can cause an infection, with itching, burning, and discharge. The most common problem is itching. Too much yeast can be fueled by a variety of things, including hormonal changes in the aftermath of taking antibiotics. Past research by Nigerian scientists show that coconut oil is effective against *Candida* strains. (Pubmed.gov: invitro Antimicrobial properties of Coconut Oil on Candida Species in Ibadan, Nigeria, Dr. D.O. Ogbulu, et. Al: 2007.)

What Oil Remedy to Use: You can use coconut oil two ways to beat a yeast infection or to prevent the onset of one. Try taking 1 tablespoon of organic virgin coconut oil three times per day for seven days. You can either add it to foods, like a smoothie, or use it as your cooking oil for stir-frys and salads. Also, applied to the site, like with the creams women can purchase without a prescription, is another method.

Why You'll Like It: For one, proponents of natural remedies will love using coconut oil because of its scent, nice and smooth texture, and most of all, because it works. A relative was anxious because she had to take a course of antibiotics. She didn't want to get a yeast infection because it would interfere with the medication she was prescribed. She opted to take coconut oil—it did its job.

Hearty Stir-Fry with Blood-Orange Olive Oil

❖ ❖ ❖

In my college days back in the twentieth century when hitchhiking was a national phenomenon, one weekend I hitchhiked to Big Sur with my roommate and black lab Stonefox. I was traveling south on the coast. It was chilly and overcast. We made two friendships—two outdoorsy men students who built a fire for us and made it a fun night. We drove together back to the San Francisco Bay Area; I offered to make a homemade meal to show appreciation. Brown rice, tofu, and vegetables—the frugal student's staple foods of the seventies. The glitch was, I got creative and added milk to give the casserole a creamy texture. When I served the dish, everyone ate, but I wish I could go back in time and create a redo. This recipe is mine, and through the years, feast or famine, I've tweaked it to perfection with a twist of oil and honey.

1 cup brown rice, cooked
1 boneless chicken breast
2 tablespoons blood-orange extra virgin olive oil
½ teaspoon fresh garlic, minced

2 tablespoons yellow onion, finely chopped
1 cup fresh cruciferous vegetables
1 Roma tomato, sliced
Ground pepper to taste

*¹/₂ cup cashews, lightly
salted, chopped
2 tablespoons honey*

*Gingersnaps
Green tea ice cream
Black tea*

Make rice according to directions. Meanwhile, wash and boil chicken till white and cooked. In a frying pan, sauté garlic and onion in olive oil and toss in cruciferous vegetables. Stir-fry for about three to five minutes. Add the cut chunks of cooked chicken. Serve on top of a bed of rice. Sprinkle with a dash of pepper. Top with cashews, and honey. For dessert, serve ginger snaps paired with all-natural green tea ice cream and black tea to give this hearty meal an Asian flair. Serves 2–3. (Double the recipe for guests or leftovers.)

THE GOLDEN SECRETS TO REMEMBER

If it doesn't specify which type of oil to use, go ahead and use your own preference: extra virgin olive oil, virgin olive oil, or other healing oils for these home cures from A to Z.

Ailment	Oil	What It May Do
Bladder infection	Olive oil, coconut oil	Soothes burning
Bruxism	Olive oil	Decreases plague
Constipation	Olive oil	Aids in regularity
Cough	Olive oil	Soothes tickle
Cuticles, dry	Olive oil, coconut oil	Heals torn skin

Ailment	Oil	What It May Do
Dandruff	Olive oil	Fights flakes
Diaper rash	Olive oil	Soothes itching and pain
Earache	Olive oil	Wards off infection and pain
Fibromyalgia	Olive oil and essential oils	Helps reduce aches and pains
Gallbladder stones	Olive oil	Soothes stomache pain
Gingivitis	Olive oil	Reduces swelling and throbbing
Hair loss	Olive oil	Aid in healthier hair and scalp
Hangover	Olive oil	Lessens headache
Hot flashes	Olive oil, flaxseed oil	Maintains normal temperature
Illness	Olive oil	Fights bacteria
Libido, lackluster	Olive oil	Revs up sex drive
Lice	Olive oil	May smother lice
Muscle aches	Almond oil, olive oil, sesame oil	Soothes pain

Ailment	Oil	What It May Do
Psoriasis	Olive oil	Gets rid of redness and scaly patches
SAD	Flaxseed oil, olive oil	Boosts energy
Skin burn Skin damage	Olive oil	Reduces pain
Sore feet	Olive oil	Eases soreness
Stomachache	Olive oil	Soothes intestinal tract
Sunburn	Coconut oil, olive oil	Relieves pain
Tendonitis	Olive oil	Relaxes muscles
Toenail fungus	Olive oil	Smoothes brittle nails
Toothache	Olive oil	Provides temporary pain relief
Universal emergency	Olive oil	Acts as cure-all
Vaginal dryness	Olive oil	Provides lubrication (but see page 208 for exceptions)

PART 6

FUTURE
OLIVE OIL

Olive Oil Mania: Using Olive Oil for the Household, Kids, Pets, and Beauty

Honor to a Spaniard, no matter how dishonest,
is as real a thing as water, wine, or olive oil.
—Ernest Hemingway[1]

During my research for the original book *The Healing Powers of Olive Oil*, I discovered dozens of uses for liquid gold for home cures—not just during the Sierra wildfire I endured. One time post-winter, I pet-sat for a neighbor. On the first day, I was in heaven. In snow flurries, my Brittany, Simon, roughhoused with his pet pal, Batman, a rat terrier. While they got their endorphin high (they were active for hours), I soaked in the hot tub, and after enjoyed a bubble bath. It was much needed R & R, sort of like an olive tree during off-harvest season.

After all the exposure to snow and water, the dog duo needed a remedy for rough, dry paw pads. I didn't know where over-the-counter moisturizing creams were, so I made do with what I found in the kitchen cupboard. I rubbed a bit of olive oil (I knew it contained hydrating properties as well as anti-inflammatory) on the pooches' pads and cold, weathered noses. While watching sci-fi doomsday films, back to back, I cuddled up in front of the gas fireplace, with the two dogs sleeping. We enjoyed the olive oil home remedy that came to the rescue and provided creature comforts.

Whether olive oil is used for home cures or heart health, this powerful golden liquid is a household name in the twenty-first century. Not only can you find olive oil in the supermarket (from commercial brands to specialty types), online, and at olive oil tree mills and estates, a variety of olive oil types is cropping up in America and worldwide.

Also, while doctors use it, nutritionists tout it, and plenty of people, like you and me, love its versatility, even conventional associations such as the American Dietetic Association and American Heart Association are giving the "liquid gold" its due kudos.

OLIVE OIL STATISTICS

MAIN OLIVE OIL PRODUCING COUNTRIES

Percent of World Supply Produced	Country
36 percent	Spain
25 percent	Italy
18 percent	Greece
8 percent	Tunisia
5 percent	Turkey
4 percent	Syria
3 percent	Morocco
1 percent	Portugal

(*Source:* United Nations Conference on Trade and Development (UNCTAD), www.unctad.org/infocom)

MAIN OLIVE OIL CONSUMING COUNTRIES

Percent of World Supply Consumed	Country
30 percent	Italy
20 percent	Spain
11 percent	Other non-European countries

9 percent	Greece
8 percent	United States
5 percent	Other European countries
3 percent	Syria
2 percent	Algeria
2 percent	Morocco
2 percent	Portugal
2 percent	Tunisia

(*Source:* United Nations Conference on Trade and Development (UNCTAD), www.unctad.org/infocom)

Since I included the olive oil producing and consuming countries in the first edition, the consensus (among research companies as well as the North American Olive Oil Association) is no surprise. Olive oil love continues to dominate Mediterranean countries. But there are even more positive projections that I agree with wholeheartedly:

- Olive oil consumption continues to soar because it is the primary component of the Mediterranean diet—and people around the globe are discovering its remarkable healing benefits.
- Greece, Spain, Italy, and North America (which may be ranked as the third largest consumer in the world) remain in the forefront as consumers of liquid gold.
- Other countries, listed in the previous consumers and producers charts, are embracing the growth potential

of the versatile olive oil market for coming years, its golden promise to continue to attract people, and its demand around the world.

Although, as mentioned before, olive oil is produced mostly in the Mediterranean countries, it is consumed in Europe, America, and other countries, too, for many reasons—including the heating of the planet.

In *The Sky Is Falling! A Global Warming Survival Guide* (AuthorHouse, 2006), my co-author, Mark Jabo, and I wrote: "The coming climatic cataclysm is the new boogeyman on the block and is so serious it's going to get you, your children, and your children's children. It will also affect your second cousin, your cousin's cousin, your children's second cousins, your children's second cousins from a previous marriage, your hamster's hamster, and the clone of your hamster's clone. Whew. Did we leave anyone out?"

Yes, we did forget the sacred olive tree. According to scientists, global warming may affect British olives. Thanks to the heating of the planet (whether humans or nature is to blame), the nation's first olive grove of more than 100 olive trees has been planted in Devon, England, and may begin producing olive oil like in the Mediterranean basin within several years. So, in the future, England may be consuming more of the golden stuff.

HEALING YOUR HOME ROOM BY ROOM

While olive oil is consumed worldwide, it's also used for a variety of household chores. When I was a teenager, I always cleaned house for my mom, who was one of those working mothers. I remember we had a cleaning lady come into our home twice a month to do the heavy chores such as cleaning the shower and oven. She would use strong chemicals to clean the showers and oven.

That was back in the 1960s. Today, women and men, like you and me, prefer to use more natural stuff rather than subject our bodies, families, pets, and friends to lingering chemicals that have potential side effects.

Are Your Household Cleaners Making You Ill?

Chemical sensitivities—are they real? You bet. These toxic chemicals can and do wreak havoc on people who use them, as well as on people who are in the environment after they are used. If you can use natural cleaners, such as olive oil and vinegar, by all means do so, to avoid these ill effects. Here are seven toxic chemicals that are guaranteed to make you plug your nose or worse.

Cleaning Chemical	Found In	Potential Side Effect
Ammonia	Glass cleaners, floor cleaners, furniture polishes	Irritates the eyes, nose, lungs; causes rashes, redness
Bleach	Disinfectants, laundry bleaches, toilet bowl cleaner	Irritates the skin; when mixed with ammonia, forms a toxic gas

Cleaning Chemical	Found In	Potential Side Effect
Formaldehyde	Disinfectants, furniture polishes, detergents	Nasal stuffinesss, itchy red eyes, nausea, headache
Glycols	Degreasers, dry cleaning chemicals, floor cleaners	Irritates the skin, eyes, nose, throat
Lye	Tub and tile cleaners	When mixed with acids, can cause harmful vapors; splashed in eyes, can cause blindness
Napthalene	Air fresheners, carpet cleaners	Dangerous to breathe; can cause headaches, nausea, confusion
Petroleum distillates	Air fresheners, carpet cleaners	Dangerous to breathe; can cause headaches, nausea, confusion

(Source: The Healing Powers of Vinegar)

Here are some things you can do with olive oil and vinegar teamed with other natural ingredients such as lemon, water, and essential oils. You'll find that these mixtures can be used to clean floors, polish furniture, freshen the air, and much, much more.

Yard

- **Repel Moles.** Some folks claim olive oil can be used to keep moles away. Soak a rag with olive oil and stuff it into the mole hole. Perhaps, a strong-flavored olive oil can do the trick. It's worth a try.
- **Prevent Rust.** I recommend keeping olive oil in the garage as well as inside the home. Coating on gardening tools may prevent rusting. Also, use olive oil on snow shovels and rakes and squeaky doors indoors and outdoors.

Living Room

- **Polish Plants.** Houseplants get dull and dusty. Try spraying with a solution of water and olive oil. Not only will you have dust-free leaves, but they will shine. Plus, if you live in a cold, dry climate and mist your plants, it is as good as talking to them.
- **Dust It Dust-Free.** Don't like to dust? Try the Vinegar Institute's all-natural remedy. Mix olive oil and vinegar in a 1-to-1 ratio and polish with a soft cloth. I tried it on my entertainment center (another hand-me-down from my dad), and it is without dust, shines, and doesn't have a chemical odor.
- **Wipe Out Table Rings.** Got rings around your tables?

I have a 30-year-old wooden living room table that I adore for sentimental reasons. I noticed a teacup ring on the lower shelf. I mixed a paste of olive oil (extra virgin) and lemon juice (2 parts olive oil to 1 part lemon juice) and applied it to the area using a circular motion, let it sit briefly, and wiped it off. The ring around my table is now gone.

- **Sparkle Up Blinds.** If you want your veneer blinds to shine like they did when you first put them up, I recommend olive oil. After you dust them, wipe them with a wet cloth dipped in gentle, soapy water, rinse, and dry. Then, apply a light coat of olive oil, and polish for a brief time, until they look like new again.

- **Love Leather Furniture.** I hesitated to use olive oil on my new, pricey leather sofa, love seat, and oversized chair. But I also didn't want to purchase a product containing harsh chemicals. The Vinegar Institute recommends a solution of distilled white vinegar and linseed oil. (I recommend olive oil.) Gently rub this protector onto your favorite leather items and rub gently with a cloth.

- **Clean Candleholders**. Do you have melted wax built up on your candleholders? No problem. Mix a solution of olive oil and mild dish soap. It takes off old wax and grime, and leaves brass, ceramic, and colored metal candleholders shining brightly.

- **Lighten Up with Lamps.** In ancient times, olive oil was used as fuel for olive oil lamps. Today, you still can purchase oil lamps—all kinds—and use them in the living room. Cabin lamps are bright and radiate more light than other lamps, such as a chamber lamp (which can be taken from room to room) or a table lamp (used for ambiance to see your clean home).

Olive Oil Keeps on Burning

So, why in the world would you use an olive oil lamp in this day and age? For starters, "They are safer than candles, because the flame is enclosed. They are also more efficient and provide better light because they don't flicker as much as candles. And they don't create any smoke or odor, for those using non-electric lighting in an enclosed area if you have allergies," explains Glenda Lehman Ervin, daughter of the founder of Lehman's Lamps. But that's not all . . .

There are a variety of perks to burning olive oil in the twenty-first century. Here are five reasons why olive oil makes a great fuel, according to the booklet *I Didn't Know That Olive Oil Would Burn!* by Merry Bickers:

1. Vegetarians and animal rights folks can sleep at night knowing that olive oil is a natural, animal-free product.
2. Religious people enjoy olive oil for its traditional use.
3. Olive oil is fume-free and a much better option for people who are sensitive to the fumes from petroleum fuels.
4. If you're on a budget, olive oil is a cost-effective fuel. For lamp fuel, you can use any kind of olive oil or can buy it in bulk, which can cut the cost.
5. Olive oil as a lamp fuel is much safer than petroleum-based fuels, which can ignite into a flame. (But note, all flames can be dangerous, and none should be left unattended, especially around young children or pets.)

Dining Room

- **Buff Brass.** To keep brass looking shinier, buff knick-knacks with olive oil after cleaning them. I have a hand-me-down collection from my dad, who was also a nature lover. So, preserving his brass birds and reindeer means a lot to me. Olive oil keeps the brass from tarnishing so fast.
- **Preserve Antiques.** I also have a glass dining room table with classic wrought iron from the good old 1950s. Rubbing a bit of extra virgin olive oil onto the iron legs of the table and four chairs using a soft cloth provides a fantastic shine to this classic and preserves its worth.

Kitchen

- **Cutting Board Cleanup.** A wooden cutting board in your kitchen is a must-have, and olive oil can help to preserve it. After using it, wash it in soap and water. Dry. Then, once it is squeaky clean, wipe it with olive oil.
- **No More Rust.** Got a cast-iron frying pan? If so, chances are it's a hand-me-down. So, you want to take care of it and keep it in tip-top condition. After each time you use it, wash it, and dry it, don't forget to lightly apply olive oil to keep it rust-free and maintain its natural shine.
- **Pamper Kitchen Helpers.** Olive oil fans use the versatile home aid to add a vibrant shine to kitchen helpers such as the blender, coffeemaker, and stainless steel toaster. After you clean these items, simply spray them with a mist of olive oil and water (3 parts water to 1 part olive oil) and buff until they gleam olive oil pretty.

Bedroom

- **Dust Delights.** Wooden furniture in your bedroom? You certainly don't want to smell chemicals from furniture polish with toxins, right? If you want to keep your personal sanctuary dust-free and smelling fragrant, use a mixture of olive oil and fresh lemon juice for the bed, nightstands, framed mirror, and picture frames.

Bathroom

- **Remove Dirt on Bathroom Floors.** Got a natural bathroom floor that could use a nice shine without the buildup of wax? After I washed my low-maintenance, all-natural-looking, neutral-colored slate floor, I mixed a few drops of olive oil with fresh lemon juice and wiped the floor once again. Ah, the fragrance and shine were enough to make me vow to never use a floor wax.
- **Polish Pretty Bathroom Treasures.** To add a nice, lasting shine to the ceramic figurines often found in a bathroom, use 3 parts olive oil and 1 part water. Buff until your treasures look bright and clean.

Family Room

- **Wow Wood-Paneling Scratches.** I live in a house that was built decades ago. It has a lot of built-in cupboards, and it's wood paneled throughout, including in the family room. I use a traditional furniture polish first and then buff surface scratches with olive oil. This makes the paneling appear scratch-free.
- **Freshen Wood.** Speaking of wood paneling, I love it. To keep it looking its best, mix 1 ounce of olive oil with 2 ounces of white vinegar and 1 quart of warm water. Dampen a soft cloth with the solution and wipe the

paneling. Then, wipe with a dry, soft cloth to remove yellowing from the surface.

Home Office

- **Get a Grime Fighter.** Black picture frames in your home office? As I looked at William Shakespeare and Einstein as well as my Barnes & Noble events posters, I decided to buff the frames with olive oil. They shine and look clean.

Laundry Room

- **Good-bye to Scratchy Lingerie.** If you have cotton underpants, I recommend mixing a solution of olive oil and mild detergent. Then handwash. Say bye-bye to expensive commercial fabric softeners, which often have strange, unnatural scents.

HEALTHY KID STUFF

When I think about children, Gemma Sanita Sciabica comes to mind. On the telephone, we discussed the topic of parents cooking healthy and how that will help their children to grow up healthy. Gemma sent me a card in which she wrote: "It is a good idea to watch children's diet making sure they do not have too much cholesterol. Using olive oil more, will prevent problems later."

- **It's Time for Pizza.** So, I thought, "Kids love pizza." Rather than order a pizza from a fast-food chain, why not make it a family night and create a healthy and tasty pie with olive oil and plenty of healthy toppings so both girls and boys can bake and choose. Here is one of Gemma's delightful pizza recipes.

Pizza Dough

❖ ❖ ❖

1¼ cups water (110°)
1 package dry yeast
3½–4 cups flour
¾ teaspoon salt

¼ cup Marsala Olive Fruit
   Oil
1 egg white

In mixing bowl, add ¼ cup water and dry yeast. Let stay about 10 minutes. In another bowl, add dry ingredients. Make well in center and pour in yeast mixture, oil, remaining water, and egg white. Stir to mix into a smooth, pliable dough. On lightly floured board, knead for several minutes. Place dough back in lightly oiled bowl, cover, and put in a warm place for about 1 hour or until doubled. Turn dough out on floured board and cut into desired sizes.

Place toppings of your choice on top of dough, then leave to rise about 20 minutes or until dough is puffy. Drizzle with olive oil. Bake in 375° oven for 20–30 minutes or until crust is golden. Makes one 15-x-10-inch or two 12-inch pies.

Variation: Substitute 1 cup whole wheat, semolina, or cornmeal flour for white flour. Add ¼ cup wheat germ.

TOPPING COMBINATIONS

- Fresh tomatoes, fresh garlic, grilled vegetables, fresh herbs, and feta or Gorgonzola cheese
- Pesto (brushed on crust), provolone, ricotta cheese, Romano cheese, fresh tomatoes, roasted garlic, and grilled mushrooms
- Grilled lemon herb chicken, roasted potatoes, and dried ricotta cheese or provolone

- Fresh tomatoes, fresh or canned clams, garlic, parsley, basil, oregano, black and red hot pepper flakes, and Romano cheese

(*Source: Cooking with California Olive Oil: Treasured Family Recipes* by Gemma Sanita Sciabica)

- **It's Time for Pasta.** *Lunch Lessons'* author Ann Cooper, former executive chef of the Putney Inn in Vermont and former president and current board member of Women's Chefs and Restaurateurs, says: "Orzo is a nice little pasta that is great in salads and side dishes. We love the fresh flavors of the herbs and lemon juice. Enlist your children to help you experiment with different herbs and vegetables by asking them to come up with some of their favorite combinations. Send this to school as a side dish to a wrap sandwich. If you want to enhance the nutritional value of this salad use whole wheat orzo."

Orzo Salad

❖ ❖ ❖

1 pound orzo pasta
5 tablespoons chopped fresh oregano
5 tablespoons chopped fresh mint leaves
6 tablespoons olive oil

3 tablespoons fresh lemon juice
½ teaspoon salt
Fresh ground black pepper as needed

Cook orzo in boiling water until tender, drain, and put in a large mixing bowl. Add oregano and mint, and toss to combine. In a small bowl, combine the oil and lemon juice, and add to orzo mixture, mixing well. Season with salt and pepper. Serves 8.

Nutrition Facts
Serving Size 1 serving
Servings Per Recipe 8
Amount Per Serving

%Daily Value

Calories 175

Calories from fat 97 (55% of total cal)

Total fat 11 g	17%
Saturated fat 2 g	8%
Cholesterol 23 mg	8%
Sodium 196 mg	8%
Total Carbohydrate 18 mg	6%
Dietary Fiber 2 g	6%

Sugars 16 g

Protein 3 g

Vitamin A 39%	**Vitamin C 10%**
Calcium 7%	Iron 25%

*Percent Daily Values are based on a 2,000 calorie diet. Your daily values may be higher or lower depending upon your caloric intake.

- **It's Time for Pie.** Fun for kids doesn't have to stop in the kitchen. Do you remember playing outdoors as a child and being able to pick fresh berries, apples, or apricots from trees in an orchard or in your own backyard? While the twenty-first century might be keeping children busy at the computer, why not join them in a nature walk and gather fresh berries? Gemma told me no-roll pie crusts are not as time-consuming to make as traditional rolled pie crusts, the type my mom used to make. So, here is a non-traditional olive oil pie crust recipe that can be used for tart shells and fresh berry pies (recipe follows). Let the good times roll.

No-Roll Pie Crust
9–10 or 11 inch

❖ ❖ ❖

1½ cups flour   ½ teaspoon salt
2 tablespoons sugar   ¼ cup milk
1 teaspoon baking powder   ½ cup Marsala Olive Oil

Preheat oven to 375°. In mixing bowl, add dry ingredients and make well in center. Pour in milk and add olive oil. Stir with fork until just combined. Gather into a ball, flatten slightly, and place in bottom of 9-inch tart pan with removable bottom.

With floured fingertips, press from center out to edge. Using the bottom of a floured ¼ cup measuring cup, press dough firmly against sides of pan. Form an edge with thumb and finger, making a small rim. Pierce bottom with fork to prevent puffing during baking. Bake 15–17 minutes or until golden. Cover edge with pie crust rim or foil if browning too quickly.

Note: For a thinner 9-inch crust, remove ¼ cup dough before pressing dough into pie pan. For a 10- or 11-inch pie crust, use dough as is. I tried to change the amounts of the ingredients in this crust, but it didn't come out as good. Now I make the crust using the amounts stated and remove the ¼ cup of dough for the 9-inch crust. No one will mind your bending from tradition when you make this no-roll pie crust. It is simple, tasty, and flaky. We really like it a lot.

To make 4-inch tart shells, press about 3 tablespoons of dough into each tart pan. Bake about 10 minutes or until golden. Fill with your favorite filling fruits. (See Fresh Berry Pie below.)

(Source: Baking Sensational Sweets with California Olive Oil, by Gemma Sanita Sciabica)

Fresh Berry Pie

❖ ❖ ❖

1 cup sugar
3 tablespoons cornstarch or
tapioca flour
4 cups boysenberries (or
berries of your choice)

¼ teaspoon cinnamon
2 tablespoons lemon juice
1 olive oil pie crust dough
(double)

Mix sugar and cornstarch, and toss with berries, cinnamon, and lemon juice. Turn into pastry lined pie plate. Bake in a 425° oven 35–45 minutes or until golden brown. Makes 9-inch pie.

(*Source: Baking Sensational Sweets with California Olive Oil* by Gemma Sanita Sciabica)

Pets and Olive Oil

1 **Smooth a Pooch's Snout** Olive oil can help soothe chapped human lips, so why not use it to soothe a canine nose cracked from chilly weather? As a Lake Tahoe resident who knows what cold, dry air does to my skin, I can tell you that oil may be helpful to dogs' cold noses. My two dogs love the snow. If their paws can become dry and cracked from the cold, dry ground, why not their tender black noses?

What Oil Remedy to Use: Use a small amount of extra virgin olive oil (only the best for our pets, right?) on your dog's nose and gently massage it.

Why You'll Like It: You'll see a smooth, shiny surface. The best part is, it's natural and doesn't have a scent.

2 **Fight Ticks** Back in the good old days, when I hitchhiked across America with my black Labrador retriever Stonefox (it was a common phenomenon in the 1970s), I recall that in mountain regions, a tick or two sometimes would find their way into his coat. Looking at the rounded body of the tick would make me squirm, while my dog didn't know the difference. I'd light a match to it and pray that the tick would work its way out of my canine's fur as I lightly pulled on it. But there are better remedies.

What Oil Remedy to Use: It's less dangerous using gentle olive oil than holding a lighted match to your best friend. Plus, as *The Passionate Olive* author Carol Firenze notes, "Ticks breathe oxygen, and they can be suffocated with a coat of olive oil."[2]

Why You'll Like It: In the film *City of Angels*, Maggie (Meg Ryan), a surgeon, must remove a tick from her yellow Lab. Her doctor-boyfriend's first recommendation is alcohol. When Maggie claims she doesn't have any hospital stuff in her home, he inquires about olive oil. She offers jalapeño or rosemary. It was a dab of rosemary olive oil that was the oil of choice and did the trick to remove the tick.

3 Ice Balls Last winter, my brother would take Simon, my fun-loving pooch, for long walks in the deep, snowy field and campground. He'd bring back my long-coated orange-and-white Brittany all wet, with his foot pads and stomach sporting ice balls that would matt his fur. Into the warm shower we'd go. Isn't there an easier solution?

What Oil Remedy to Use: Firenze seems to think so. She says to fill a plastic spray bottle with olive oil and "spritz it on the fur" to zap the ice and snow and smooth the fur. My first reaction was "No way!" I've witnessed these thick ice balls, and warm water does the trick. However, spraying olive oil on a dog's coat afterwards is a good idea, since it keeps the fur soft and conditioned.[3]

Why You'll Like It: Naturally, it would be a godsend if Firenze's remedy worked. Note to self: Spray extra virgin olive oil (nothing but the best for my two boys) on their coats next snow day. However, I will have fresh towels ready for warm-water applications or a shower just in case. P.S.: I will also use that olive oil spritz on my hands, to keep them soft after tending to the dogs.

4 **Gooey Foot Pads** Uh-oh. Did Fluffy or Fido step in something sticky such as gum or tar? This sticky situation can be frustrating for both pet and caretaker. So, what can you do rather than watch your poor cat or dog lick and chew the unwanted substance? Olive oil comes to the rescue.

What Oil Remedy to Use: Try soaking the foot pad in a solution of warm saltwater and olive oil. The two ingredients may break up the foreign substance, and both the oil and the salt may also soothe any redness.

Why You'll Like It: Using a natural salt–olive oil solution may do the trick, especially if the substance doesn't cover the entire foot pad. If it works, it beats cutting the fur, ignoring the situation, or watching your companion animal struggle to make it better while it only gets worse. Plus, a home cure that gets a thumbs-up is preferred to a pricey vet visit.

5 **Clean Ears** Dogs and cats can get ear mites, small parasitic creatures that take up residence in their ears, causing itching and inflammation. Olive oil or a natural product that contains it, whether you use it to prevent a case of ear mites or to treat it, may help ease the itch and fight the infection.

What Oil Remedy to Use: Firenze recommends olive oil because it will "drown the mites." You can dab olive oil on a cotton ball and rub gently inside and outside your pet's ear canal. Or, you can use an olive oil–based natural pet product for ear mites.[4]

Why You'll Like It: Well, it's natural. And if it does work, it is better than ignoring the problem and then having to pay a professional to treat it when it becomes a pesky problem that neither you nor your pet can tune out.

6 **Cancer Fighter** Cats and dogs over 10 years of age (and even younger) can receive the earth-shattering diagnosis of cancer. But as frightened as they may become, I know pet lovers are not powerless. When my 18-year-old cat developed cancer, surgery bought him more time. But pets, like people, can also take advantage of a holistic arsenal—herbs, homeopathy, natural nutrition, and dietary supplements—to prevent and treat cancer.

What Oil Remedy to Use: Add olive oil to your pet's diet. It will help prevent free-radical damage to cells, which can lead to abnormal cell growth. Consult with a holistic veterinarian regarding the amount, since it will vary depending on the weight of the cat or dog.

Why You'll Like It: Using natural cancer fighters like olive oil in your pet's daily diet regimen will help you be proactive.

7 **Canine Chow** A devout olive oil fan who calls herself "The Garden Lady" told me, "Olive oil should be in everyone's dog dish." She insists it makes her dog's coat shiny, "and he thinks he's getting 'people food.' I

make a production of taking the bottle off the counter that's next to the stove, so he knows that he's getting some of our provisions. The plain chow he won't eat, but the chow with olive oil is absolutely inhaled."

What Oil Remedy to Use: Put 1 teaspoon of olive oil in your dog's food daily. Note: Consult with your veterinarian first to make sure the amount is appropriate for your pet, since the weight of a 5-pound teacup poodle is different than that of a large Labrador retriever.

Why You'll Like It: If you go to a holistic vet, chances are olive oil will get a thumbs-up. However, a conventional vet may tell you that there is no reason to include the oil in your pet's diet or may suggest a commercial brand of essential fatty acids to add to your dog's food.

8 **Dog and Cat Shampoo** Ever consider adding olive oil to your pet's shampoo? It's not unheard of, at all. The olive oil may keep the skin healthy and leave the coat shining, according to people who make and/or use the oil in pet grooming products. Also, it may help maintain good skin hydration and even prevent matting on a long-haired canine.

What Oil Remedy to Use: Mix 1/2 teaspoon with your pet's recommended amount of natural shampoo. Massage in, then rinse.

Why You'll Like It: If you're like me, you may prefer to use olive oil topically on your pet rather than to include it in your pet's food. It's a quick, all-natural way to keep your dog's coat looking good and feeling great. Note: I did massage a dab of olive oil into Simon's dry coat (like I did for my own hair) and followed with a brushing. The outcome: His coat appeared a bit on the oily side. The second day, it looked like he was having a good canine hair day.

9 **Use Natural Dog Treats** Want to give your dog (or cat) a special edible treat but don't want chemicals? No problem. In fact, did you know that there are natural products on the market that actually contain olive oil?

What Oil Remedy to Use: Most supermarkets don't have a wide selection of natural pet treats, but if you're lucky (read the labels), you may find one or two brands. I purchased one brand at the grocery store, and it contained canola oil.

Why You'll Like It: If you don't like eating foods with chemicals and preservatives, you probably want to feed your pets all-natural goodies, too. Once you find a brand they like, you'll be pleased to know that it's a good and healthful snack for your animal angels. Or, if you want to be sure your critters get olive oil–based treats, you can make them yourself.

10 **Make Olive Oil Goodies** Wish you had an easy-to-bake dog biscuit recipe? Online, you'll find a variety of homemade pet treats, and in some natural pet-care books, you'll also find recipes that include olive oil.

What Oil Remedy to Use: I suggest using extra virgin olive oil because you want to give the best to your best friend, right? Some recipes call for 2 tablespoons of olive oil.

Why You'll Like It: "We use olive oil because it is such an excellent source of omega fatty acids, and typically, in the diet of today's dog, essential fatty acids (EFAs) are sadly lacking," say the dog experts at www.knowbetterdogfood.com. Plus, vets will tell you that if your dog's coat lacks shine, your companion animal may be lacking EFAs.

Adds the Two Dog Press expert: "We use olive oil in our treat recipes because I use olive oil almost exclusively in my cooking for humans. It's what I always have available in the cupboard. Plus, it's a rich source of good, healthy, vegetable-based fat and it adds more flavor than corn or safflower oils."

Dog Biscuits They'll Roll Over For!

❖ ❖ ❖

Big Boy Beef Biscuits

½ cup dry milk
1 egg
1 teaspoon parsley
6 tablespoons olive oil
2 teaspoons honey
1 small (2.5-ounce) jar beef baby food

½ cup beef broth
1 cup whole wheat flour
½ cup rye flour
½ cup rice flour
½ cup cracked wheat

GLAZE
1 egg
2 tablespoons beef broth

Preheat oven to 325°. In a large bowl, combine the dry milk, egg, parsley, oil, honey, baby food, and broth. Gradually blend in the flours and cracked wheat. Add enough wheat flour to form a stiff dough. Transfer to a floured surface and knead until smooth, about 3–5 minutes. Shape the dough into a ball and roll to 1/2-inch thick. Using bone-shaped cookie cutters, make biscuits. Transfer to ungreased baking sheets, spacing about 1/4 inch apart. Gather up the scraps, roll out again, and cut additional biscuits. Bake for 30 minutes. Whisk together the egg and broth for the glaze. Brush biscuits with the glaze on both sides. Return to oven and bake for an additional 30 minutes. Let cool overnight.

Makes several dozen small bones or 2½–3 dozen large bones, depending on the size of the cookie cutter.

(*Courtesy:* Two Dog Press http://www.twodogpress.com/dog food.html)

Now that we've put popular olive oil on the table and explained how to use it to make a happy home and maintain healthy kids and pets, take a look at how the versatile oil—either by itself or as an ingredient in ready-made beauty products—can help to beautify you from head to toe.

Macadamia Nut Oil Pumpkin Cake

❖ ❖ ❖

2 extra large organic brown   1 premium spice cake mix*
   eggs   1 cup water
4 tablespoons grass-fed   2 tablespoons macadamia
   butter   nut oil

*Look at the ingredients label on the cake mix. Try to avoid products listing trans fats or partially hydrogenated oil.

1 cup canned pumpkin
   puree
1 teaspoon pumpkin spice
1 teaspoon ground cin-
   namon

¾ cup dark chocolate chips
Sugar in the raw, 100 percent natural turbindo
   cane
European-style butter

Butter a Bundt pan or square dish with European-style butter and set aside. In a mixing bowl, beat eggs and melted butter. Stir in cake mix and flour. Add water, oil, and pumpkin puree. Sprinkle in pumpkin spice and cinnamon and stir. Fold in chocolate chips. Mix until batter is smooth without lumps. Using large spatula, put batter into pan; smooth so it's flat. Bake at 350° for 40 minutes or till a knife inserted in the middle of the cake comes out clean and is firm to touch. Cool for 10 minutes, then place a plate on top and turn over. Cool and sprinkle with raw sugar.

THE GOLDEN SECRETS TO REMEMBER

- ✓ Spain, Italy, and Greece are the top olive oil producing countries in the world as well as the top consumers.
- ✓ Olive oil can be used to heal your home in a variety of amazing ways.
- ✓ If you have chemical sensitivities or care about using eco-friendly cleaning products inside and outside your home, olive oil is the choice for you.
- ✓ It's never too soon to teach your kids how to eat and cook healthy. Olive oil can help you do just that.
- ✓ Olive oil is an all-purpose natural remedy for both cats and dogs that can provide better health and edible treats.

Olive Beautiful

His branches shall spread, and his beauty shall be as the olive tree.

—Bible[1]

Taking care of companion animals by using olive oil as a home cure is one thing, but discovering its multipurpose beauty pluses is another experience worth sharing. While I love a mountain environment, it comes with lack of humidity, sun damage, wind, and snow, which all can wreak havoc on your skin from head to toe.

One afternoon, I was tending the rustic front deck, sweeping and arranging potted plants. Without any foreshadowing, something tore open the bottom of my foot. I looked down at the weathered brown wood, and I saw the culprit. I stepped on a rusty, protruding nail—it punctured my skin. The pain was excruciating; but the thought of getting a tetanus shot was now on my mind.

Since it was a Sunday, I paid a visit to the clinic, not my own general practitioner. The nurse gave me advice about my dry feet as she was cleaning the bottom of them. She recommended different over-the-counter remedies, such as Vaseline, while the doctor cut the torn skin on my clean foot. One shot later, I made some resolutions. I vowed to wear shoes on the deck, and I began to use olive oil on my feet to keep them soft. I even rubbed the oil on my sunburned arms and legs, hoping its healing compounds would soothe the ache from the injection site as well as the redness on my shoulders.

The only thing better than pampering your home and pets is spoiling yourself. When I was a kid, my grandmother allowed us to take deep, lukewarm bubble baths in the middle of hot summer days. She'd bring in snacks for us to nibble on, from cold cuts, which included fresh carrots, celery, cherry tomatoes, and both black and green olives, and tall glasses of iced tea.

Today, spa resorts and day spas offer a variety of pampering treats. But you can get the same benefits right at home. A bathtub (or shower), quality time, and the right olive oil–based cosmetics and soaps are all you need.

Olive oil itself and ready-made products come in the form of bath oil, body gel, hand lotion, lip balm, shampoo, crème rinse, and soap. Thanks to my research, I've tried each and every one of them. And because I'm a natural woman, I am hooked on the magic of olive oil for beauty.

For centuries, Mediterranean women have turned to olive oil to condition their hair, making it shine. Italian actress Sophia Loren, at 71, told the media that the secret to her youthful looks is "the odd bath in virgin olive oil." Olive oil has been used for skin treatments since biblical times—and in the twenty-first century, it's finding its way back as a beauty product around the world.

While women and men have countless beauty products to

use, I decided to try some ready-made olive oil–based soaps to see if they are worth the "gold" that the oil once was in historical times.

THE OLIVE AND THE BEAUTY

Shampoos and Conditioners:
Baronessa Cali Body Building Shampoo
Baronessa Cali Conditioner

These were part of a gift. I used both. I do have my favorite shampoos (the kind that promise full and thick hair), but I confess these products with "extracts of Italian Olive Oil" left my hair soft (yes, incredibly silky) and nice to touch, while my curly locks are prone to dryness in the winter months and due to the chlorine from swimming in both indoor and outdoor pools year round.

Olive Oil Lotions and Gels:
Baronessa Cali Hand and Body Moisturizer
Baronessa Cali Shower and Bath Gel

I am in love with my Cali hand and body lotion. The torn cuticles on my hands every winter are nonexistent this time around. In the morning and at night at work in my study, I use it religiously. Plus, I prefer a natural-based hand and body lotion rather than one with ingredients I can't pronounce. So, without doubt, this Cali lotion works for me.

I don't often use gels in the shower, but it is a treat to do so. It's something I will do if I go to a spa or when I travel and pamper myself at a plush hotel. So, to be able to use a product like this, and a natural good-for-you one, is a treat, and like the other Cali products, it made my skin feel smooth, clean, and pampered.

The Man Behind
Extra Virgin Olive Oil Soaps

Who in the olive oil world makes and sells only olive oil soaps? Meet Elie Maghames, a charming Lebanon-born man who grew up in France. In America for nearly 20 years, he opened up the olive oil store L'Olivier in Sonoma, California, in 2001. The ambitious entrepreneur sold fifty types of olive oils and vinegars. By 2004, he noticed it was his olive oil soaps that were the moneymakers.

"After tasting all of the olive oil, we didn't like some, and we thought they weren't good enough for our customers, so we started making olive oil soap," points out Maghames. A few months passed, and they provided only ten fragrances, while there were daily requests to add more scents. Nowadays, L'Olivier has about eighty fragrances. Many of these soaps are made with extra virgin olive oil.

Some of the natural essential oil fragrances include: grapefruit, lime, lavender, lavender/clove/orange, lavender/ lime, lavender/eucalyptus/tea tree, oatmeal/lavender/peppermint, orange, patchouli, and rosemary/sage.

These days, you can find Maghames selling only soaps and skin care products, such as olive oil soaps, olive massage oils, lip salves, and specialty soaps. In fact, his business is growing, so he will be relocating to a larger, factory-type building to continue his work.

With a French accent and down-to-earth manner, Maghames freely talks about his products and their unique qualities. He believes olive oil is one of the few oils that goes deep into the skin without clogging the pores. It attracts moisture to the skin and prevents it from drying.

"Growing up around the Mediterranean Sea, I

was amazed to see ladies of all ages using olive oil on their hair and skin daily. Their hair was fluffy and healthy, and their bodies were very soft. My grandma used to tell me: 'If the oil can protect inside your body, why not the outside,'" recalls Maghames.

BEAUTY TIPS FROM HEAD TO TOE

Ready-made products are a treat because they're convenient and smell nice. But, using olive oil by itself or with other ingredients from your kitchen cupboards can work wonders, too. In fact, using both olive oil out of a bottle and ready-made olive oil–based soaps and skin care products is like having the best of both worlds. Go ahead—try using olive oil solo for your crowning glory to your tender feet.

- **Soft and Shiny Hair.** Fatty acid–rich olive oil can penetrate the hair cuticle and smooth dry hair. Celebrity hairstylists and beauty experts recommend putting a few drops of olive oil in the palm of your hand and rubbing until the skin glistens. Then, work the oil into your locks, starting at the ends.

  I did this months ago—first with canola oil and then with extra virgin olive oil. Both oils do the trick. Your hair, especially if it's exposed to a cold, dry climate, chlorine, blow dryers, curling irons, or hair products, will be softer and silkier to touch, and it will appear less dry and have a nice sheen.

- **Hair Conditioner.** Looking for a deep conditioning treatment for dry hair? Combine ¼ cup extra virgin olive oil with $\frac{1}{4}$ cup spring water. Massage into your dry hair, and cover with a plastic bag. Wait 20 minutes, shampoo, and use your regular hair conditioner.

- **Skin Moisturizer.** Many women have told me that they use extra virgin olive oil on their hair and face at night as a moisturizer. In the morning, I use an all-purpose moisturizing crème with SPF 15. At night, I use the olive oil nighttime remedy. I apply the oil to my face, around my eyes, and on my laugh lines (and the extra I rub into my hands and cuticles). In the morning, my skin feels softer than usual. A bonus: Antiaging crèmes cost $15 and up. This remedy costs less—and may do more.

- **Eye Makeup Remover.** If you wear eyeliner, mascara, and eye shadow, like women do to enhance their eyes, you also know that it is a task to remove these beauty enhancers. An easy-does-it eye makeup remover may be as close to you as your kitchen cabinet.

  Try mixing 1 tablespoon of canola oil with 1 tablespoon of extra virgin olive oil. Apply a small amount to a cotton ball and wipe your eyelashes and eyelids.

- **Smooth Shaving Cream.** Olive oil fans insist the oil can be used to shave. Not only does it moisturize, but it will soften the hair and make the procedure more comfy for a man's beard or woman's legs. Try mixing 1 tablespoon of extra virgin olive oil, $\frac{1}{2}$ cup of warm water, and 1 tablespoon of a gentle liquid soap. For best results, use a clean, sharp razor.

- **Soften Elbows.** In the spring and summertime, it's common to notice rough elbows. But why not take care of this alligator-type skin year-round? Then, whether it's shower time or bedtime, you'll have one less beauty woe.

Italy's Antonio recommends his grandmother's easy-to-do remedy. Dip your elbows in a bowl of lukewarm olive oil. (Warm it up in the microwave.) Repeat as needed, and your elbows will become smooth before you can say "soft elbows."

- **Stretch Marks.** Both women and men can get those small, depressed streaks in the skin that appear on the tummy, buttocks, thighs, hips, and breasts. While they are most common on the stomach in the later stages of pregnancy when the belly is quickly expanding, they also can be seen on people who gain weight (or build up muscle) and lose body fat or muscle mass rapidly. Plus, if your mom or dad had stretch marks, you may, too, thanks to the genetic factor.

  To minimize those marks on your body, rub olive oil on the area at least twice daily. When celebrity Brooke Burke had to have a bikini-ready body a few months after childbirth for a photo shoot, she turned to oil during her pregnancy, according to Celebrity Parents (www.celebrityparents.com). "I rubbed oil into my hips, belly and breasts every day, twice a day," she says. "You can use shea butter, cocoa butter, almond oil, or any natural oil. It's really essential."

- **Sexy Feet.** Kris, a genuine olive oil lover, swears by olive oil for making her feet soft. "On an evening when you can soak your feet," she says, she does it, and she goes the whole 9 yards. "I rub olive oil to treat rough skin, then put on some thick socks. You can leave that on overnight. For a real soft foot treatment, soak those feet in vinegar first, then rub with olive oil and your feet will be baby soft."

TUB TIME

Bathing with olive oil is nothing new. Centuries ago, the Romans and the Egyptians used olive oil for moisturizing during and after tub time. By the nineteenth century, bathing for pleasure was a popular pastime in Europe and the word "spa" was created.

Some people claim that using a few drops of olive oil in a bath is a great natural moisturizer. But note, if you are prone to bladder infections or vaginal infections, contact your doctor before you take a dip and ask for a thumbs-up on using soothing olive oil combined with natural essential oils. (If it isn't recommended or if you don't have a bathtub, try plan B: Take a shower and use ready-made soaps with olive oil and essential oils.)

For best results, follow these suggestions straight from aromatherapy experts: Put specific essential oils on the skin before getting into the bath, light a scented candle or two for a sensual effect, and indulge in a cup of calming chamomile tea while you soak and beautify yourself.

Olive Oil and Scented Bath	Benefit	Essential Oil
Wake-up	Invigorates	Peppermint, rosemary
Foot soak	Relieves tired feet and athlete's foot	Witch hazel, tea tree
Aches	Relieves muscle soreness	Eucalyptus, lemon
De-stress	Relieves stress	Chamomile, orange
Insomnia	Promotes sleep	Lavender, chamomile

Using olive oil at home to pamper yourself is one thing, but traveling to a luxury spa and being pampered with olive oil is heaven—or it seems to be.

At the Napa Valley Lodge, California, the spa offers one beauty treatment, "Olive You." This is a massage/scalp and hair/foot treatment. The online description reads: "Your whole body, skin, hair and feet are cared for in this popular treatment. Your feet are scrubbed with olive oil, apricot kernels and peppermint oil and snugly wrapped to open the pores. Then we hydrate your feet with soothing balm . . . Finish with a grape seed/olive oil massage." The cost: $150 for a 90-minute treatment.

Or, at Carneros Inn in Napa, you can indulge in an "orchard olive stone and honeydew exfoliation. A unique exfoliation of warm crushed olive stones mixed with our native Carneros olive oil, followed by a luxurious massage with a rich honeydew body cream." The cost: $100 for a 45-minute treatment.

Now that you've got olive oil beauty secrets down, from head to toe, it's time to meet the real live people behind this liquid gold and the people who travel on the olive oil trail. We'll talk one-on-one with some unique people who make olive oil, as well as with folks who travel thousands of miles, to Sonoma, California, and Tuscany, Italy, to tour and taste olive oils.

Sesame Crisps

❖ ❖ ❖

Crisp and crunchy, nutty with the taste of sesame, these saucer-sized ultra-thin crackers are a snap to make, and teamed with hummus or baba ghanoush, make a wonderful hors d'oeovre. Try them with tabbouleh or another summer salad, or just enjoy as is with a cool twilight drink.

1½ cups (6 ounces) Italian flour or pastry flour
⅓ cup (2¾ ounces) water
2 tablespoons (⅞ ounce) olive oil
¾ teaspoon salt
½ cup (2½ ounces) sesame seeds, toasted

Combine all the ingredients to make a stiff dough. You can do this by hand, with the help of an electric mixer, or in a bread machine set on the manual cycle. Knead the dough for a minute or less; you don't need to develop the gluten, just make sure all of the ingredients are thoroughly combined. Shape the dough into a flattened ball, cover it with plastic wrap, and set it aside to rest and relax at room temperature for 15 minutes.

Divide the dough into eight equal pieces, each about the size of a golf ball (1¼ to 1½ ounces each). Roll each piece into a ball, then flatten the balls. Cover them and let rest for 15 minutes.

Preheat the oven to 425° . If you have a baking stone, place it on the floor of your gas oven or on the lowest rack of your electric oven. If you don't have a baking stone, place a cookie sheet on the lowest rack of the oven.

Transfer the dough to a lightly greased work surface. Working with one piece at a time, roll the dough into a thin, 6-inch-wide circle. Set the circle aside and continue rolling the dough until you've got eight thin rounds.

Working quickly, pick up two pieces of dough and gently toss them onto the baking stone or baking sheet, making sure they lie flat. Close the oven door and bake for 3 minutes. Using a spatula or tongs, turn the rounds over and bake for 3 minutes on the other side, until the rounds are a light golden brown on the edges. (Check them after 2 to 2½ minutes to be sure they're not too brown; they can burn quickly.) Remove the crisps from the oven and quickly spray or brush them with garlic or sesame oil. Place on rack to cool. Repeat with the remaining rounds. Eat immediately or store in airtight container.

(*Courtesy: The King Arthur Flour Baker's Companion: The All-Purpose Baking Cookbook*)

THE GOLDEN SECRETS TO REMEMBER

✓ Olive oil–based ready-made products include bath oils, body gels, hand lotions, and shampoos.
✓ It takes special people to make special olive oil beauty products for people to enjoy.

✓ Olive oil from the bottle can condition your hair and skin—in or out of the tub—and be used to soften your body from your elbows to your feet.
✓ Remember, team olive oil with fragrant essential oils to double the effect and get health benefits, too.
✓ Olive oil treatments at luxury spas can be a treat to your senses.

Olive Oil Producers, Tasting Bars, and Tours

Good oil, like good wine, is a gift from the gods.
—George Ellwanger[1]

This time around when revisiting Olive Oil Land, I received new olive oil–infused beauty products from Baronessa Cali Cosmetics. If olive trees could be humanized, I'm sure they would be proud if shown the end results of what they produce. The array of items, including body scrub and face cream, had me at presentation (the packaging truly is awesome with its earthy green color and dark olives), and each one wooed me with its nature-based compounds.

While olive oil, straight from the bottle, works beautifying wonders, I was eager to pamper myself with ready-made wonders in attractive boxes, bottles, and tubes. It was to be a head-to-toe experience; and now I'm addicted. Here's why.

One morning at 7:30 A.M., during off-season, a time when our ski resort town is empty with no tourists and simply locals, I pampered myself with the array of olive oil beauty products. After my swim and hot tub, I headed to the women's room, complete with sauna and steam rooms. I fantasized that I was all alone—no dogs waiting eagerly for me at home—at a health spa resort far away in a European country. Then, I used product after product, and after each one, enjoyed the morphing of my body inside and outside. It was a weekday to cherish, and I even enjoyed images of one of the Baronessa's historical moments that whisked my imagination away to Europe . . .

As the story goes, in a Sicilian town, her great-great-grandfather Gesualdo Di Naro made a great find. As an olive and orange grove farmer (much like my dream I discussed in Chapter 1), he discovered an orange with a distinct color, later called "Tarocco," aka "blood orange." Thus, the antioxidant-rich fruit has been used by her family both inside and outside the body with promise of keeping the skin soft. Needless to add, when I used and use these items with Italian roots, my mind and senses go abroad without leaving my cozy Californian home.

During the research and writing the first edition of this book, it was fall, in the height of harvest season. Also, September 23 is the day celebrated for the olive tree. As a Libra, born on October 6, this is my favorite time of year. I can attest, however, that many olive oil producers were not favorable, at first, to my calls when I contacted them. I felt like a pesky intruder barging in at the wrong time, right place. For example, when I asked one woman the question "Which olive ranch is the largest in California?" she snapped, "Count the trees." But I pondered, "There has to be an easier way to determine which olive oil producers are successful." So, I put on my reading glasses and did my homework, both at home and at the olive oil orchards. (Just kidding.)

I soon discovered many of the olive oil producers and the

manufacturers of olive oil–based products resided in Northern California, my home. And, many of them extended a warm Indian Summer welcome to me despite their grueling schedule to tend to their early or late harvest of olive oil.

EARLY AND LATE OLIVE HARVESTS

Fall Harvest Olive Oil: Olives reach their full size in the fall but may not fully ripen from green to black until late winter. Green olives have slightly less oil and more bitterness and can be higher in disease-fighting polyphenols. The oil tends to be more pricey because it takes more olives to make one bottle.

Many people like the peppery and bitter qualities of early-harvest oil. I like the former but pass on the latter, although it may just take a while to savor it, like getting used to goldenseal tea. Flavor notes of *astringent, grass, green, green leaf,* and *pungent* are used to describe early-harvest oils. Because of the higher polyphenols and antioxidants, early-harvest oils often have a longer shelf life and are blended with late-harvest oils to improve their shorter shelf life.

Winter Harvest Olive Oil: The fruit is picked black and ripe. The fruit may have a little more oil, but waiting to harvest it is risky business because as the days get shorter, the longer nights rev up the risk of the fruit being damaged by unwanted frost.

Late-harvest or "winter" fruit is naturally more ripe, so like other ripe fruit (think of a banana sitting on top of your refrigerator one day too many), it has a light, mellow taste with little bitterness and more floral flavors. Flavor notes of *apple, banana, buttery, fruity, melon, peach, perfumy, rotund, soave,* and *sweet* are often used.

Spring Harvest Olive Oil: Early March through late April is the last time to pick and press olives before the next season rolls around. These olives are ripe with a capital "R" and black on black all the way through to the pit. Olive oil from this season is the most delicate and "buttery sweet" available, dubbed "Limited Release" by California's Sciabica family due to its scarcity.

(*Source: The Olive Oil Source* and Sciabica)

THE PRODUCERS

As I sit in my Northern California study, I confess that it didn't seem practical to book a flight to Europe and count the trees or acres to determine which producers are yielding the most olive oil. That would be a job in itself. And, in years to come, the number of trees and acres will change, from estate to estate, just as they do in California. But one man did do the legwork worldwide, so to speak. Charles Quest-Ritson provides impressive statistics about producers of olive oil in his book *Olive Oil*. The numbers will give you an idea. Here, take a look:

- **Spain.** Spain is touted as the largest olive-producing country worldwide. "It has more than 300 million olive trees covering more than five million acres, 92 percent of which are grown for olive oil," notes Quest-Ritson. Also, Jaen province produces a large percentage, and Martos is important. It claims to be the "World Capital of olive oil."[2]
- **Italy.** This country produces approximately 555,000 to 777,000 tons on a yearly basis. Nearly half of the total comes from Puglia, in southern Italy. Calabria, Sicily, and Campania follow.[3]

- **Greece.** These days, the total region planted with olives, says Quest-Ritson, is more than 2.4 million acres, with about 150 million olive trees, 2,800 mills, and more than 100 olive cultivars. What's more, Greece makes about 440,000 tons of oil each year.[4]

WIDESPREAD OLIVE APPEAL

While Spain, Italy, and Greece are known as the front-runners of olive oil production, other countries around the world are not ignoring olive oil. In China to Northern California, olive oil producers are showing enthusiasm with their orchards, mills, and olive oil.

Northern California is also becoming popular with the olive oil industry, with olive oil estates, tours, and tastings.

It is a competitive olive oil world, I learned. As a devout and serious dog person who used to breed Labrador retrievers and is now owned by two purebred Brittanys, I understand the ranking of and awards for dogs. It is similar in the world of olive oils. There are award-winning oils, judges, and tastings, and, well, olive oils can be ranked just like show dogs in a national or international show ring. And it's amazing to live in the Golden State where award-winning olive oils are produced.

California Olive Oil—In Perspective

Paul Vossen of the University of California, Davis, has a handle on the California olive oil industry. Here's his outlook on California, which is the only state with significant production:

In 2006, California produced an estimated 400,000 gallons of olive oil, which is only 0.06% of the world's olive oil and less than 1% of the USA's domestic consumption of about 60 million gallons. . . .

Most of the 10,200 estimated acres of olive oil orchards in California have been planted in the last ten years; about 40% in just the last two years. Most of the older orchards that went in at the start of the gourmet olive oil resurgence in the late 1980s and early 1990s were planted in coastal counties. They are growing primarily Italian cultivars such as Frantoio, Leccino, Maurino, and Pendolino. Most of the newest plantings are located in the Central Valley with the varieties Arbequina, Arbosana, and Koroneiki. . . . When the currently planted acreage in California comes into bearing over the next 3–5 years, the state will be producing 1 million gallons of olive oil per year.

California's olive oils, as defined by flavor and style, have been closely associated with variety, harvest maturity, and processing technique. Many examples of California olive oils produced in the coastal counties, the Sierra foothills, and in Central Valley orchards have won awards internationally.

OLIVE OIL TASTING SMARTS

Here are several common terms you will hear aficionados use when judging the flavor of an olive oil.

Good Stuff	Bad Stuff
Almond: nutty	Bitter: good in moderation, but bad if overwhelming
Bitter: preferred trait of olive oils; often from green olives	Dirty: retains the unpleasant odor and flavor of its vegetable water, with which it remained in contact too long after pressing
Fresh: good aroma, fruity	Earthy: a musty humid odor from being pressed from unwashed, muddy olives
Grass: grass-like taste, common in green olives or those crushed with leaves and twigs	Flat: no aroma, tasteless
Green: young, fresh, fruity	Frozen: made from olives that weathered freezing temperatures; unpleasant odor
Peppery: a peppery bite in the back of the throat that causes a cough	Greasy: a grease flavor

Good Stuff	Bad Stuff
Pungent: a burning sensation in the throat	Musty: moldy taste from being stored too long before pressing
Sweet: not bitter or pungent; common in mellow oils	Rancid: old; has begun to oxidize because of exposure to light or air

(*Source:* John Deane, M.D.)

OLIVE OIL TOUR DIARY: FORCES OF NATURE IN THE GOLDEN STATE

DAY ONE

As luck would have it, Murphy's Law is haunting me on November 28. As a resident of South Lake Tahoe, I shouldn't be surprised that Mother Nature would hinder our planned trip to "oliveland"—just three and a half hours away. A snowstorm is on its way, and it's wreaking havoc on our schedule to go to The Olive Press, Round Pond, B.R. Cohn, and Frantoio's. Well, we will visit all four hot olive oil spots—but not on the designated timetable.

One day late, at 4:10 P.M., my best friend, Kim Barrow, my younger brother, Bruce, and my two fun-loving Brittanys arrive intact near Round Pond in Rutherford, California. No snow in sight. I see a breathtaking Mediterranean type of terrain. The temperature is mild outdoors at the olive mill where oil is extracted from picked olives for Round Pond, a family-owned business that also makes vinegars and wines.

Amid the olive trees and European landscape, this mill

sitting in Napa Valley is picture-perfect to me, a native of the Bay Area still trying to adapt to cold mountain weather, I think as I introduce myself to Round Hill's gracious tour director, who gives us a tour of the Rutherford oil mill.

She explains that Miles and Ryan MacDonnell, the owners, live on the premises, with some 2,100 trees in their 12-acre orchard. I am envious. It is so different from my mountain lifestyle, with pine trees surrounding my cabin, which sits a few blocks from Lake Tahoe. I feel like I am in another country—a European place.

The guide shows us two of the mills. One has granite wheels to crush the olives. These are the best to play up the mellow Spanish-style oils. The other is a hammer mill to mince the olives into a pulp, best for Italian-style oils. Also, our tour guide emphasizes, time is of the essence—48 hours is the time for picking and crushing. No longer. This isn't vinegar; it's artisanal olive oil.

Inside a small room, Kim and I follow our guide, who has an elegant table laid out for us, her two olive oil–tasting guests. A variety of olive oils are sitting in front of us surrounded by good-for-you edibles such as leafy lettuce, cheese, French bread, and red wine vinegar. Kim is bold and tastes each and every olive oil—the way it's supposed to be done. I make myself a salad and splash vinegar and olive oil on it. Not the right way to taste and judge, but it works for me. We thank our hostess and leave, realizing that olive oil is a serious business and there is a time to harvest and a time to reap. And our tour would have been longer if we had been on time, I think to myself.

It is back on the road, this time to Mill Valley. I have a 7:30 P.M. interview with Dr. Roberto Zecca, former owner of Frantoio's Restaurant and the former president of the California Olive Oil Council. Once at the location, we check in at the Holiday Inn Express, chosen for its convenience and pet-friendly policy. (Rome, Italy, also has a pooch-friendly Holiday Inn, I recall.)

I choose to go solo for my interview. As I walk toward the restaurant, which boasts a terra-cotta–toned exterior, I fantasize I am in Italy, a place I will go to one day. Inside, I am told by the hostess that Dr. Zecca had a family emergency and therefore won't be able to make our interview date. Disappointed, I gaze around me and admire the high ceilings, stone floors, and built-in booths. I don't want to leave. Then, the general manager comes to my rescue.

I am whisked off to my own booth with a full view of the oakwood-fired oven. To the left of me, I also get to view Frantoio's state-of-the-art olive press—behind a gigantic piece of glass at the back of the busy restaurant. It has huge granite wheels, used to grind the olives to paste. This particular night, the press is down. (The olive press has since been replaced by a horizontal decanter centrifuge.) Still, I get a tour (and you can get a virtual one at www.frantoio.com) and am impressed that the restaurant makes its own extra virgin olive oil on-site. Plus, I later discover, Frantoio also provides custom presses for more than two dozen clients. It's unique, and so is the house-made extra virgin olive oil used in all of its dishes.

The menu boasts seasonal Tuscan delights using local produce and cheeses. I select the margherita brick-oven pizza, made with San Marzano tomatoes, mozzarella, basil, and extra virgin olive oil. As I sip chamomile tea, I dip homemade bread (with olives) into freshly made extra virgin olive oil. (Yes, for me, this is an adventure.)

Then, former chef Duilio Valenti, a 30-something friendly man from Milan, pays a visit to my table. Not only are the pizza and service delightful, the ambiance is warm, casual, and comfortable.

Once I make my way back to the hotel, I am greeted by Kim, Bruce, and my two dogs. They ordered in from Frantoio's menu and I get a taste of more Italian cuisine: tortelloni filled with Pino's fresh ricotta and swiss chard with walnut sauce and olio novella, as well as more homemade bread. For dessert, Torre di Chioccolato, we indulge in a moist Valrhona chocolate cake tower. We are content with the chef's culinary skills.

DAY TWO

While my trip to the Valley of the Moon is an unforgettable one, it by no means is unique. Countless people visit olive oil spots, just like the two characters in the film *Sideways*, who go on a wine-tasting road trip.

I admit, due to the snowstorm, we are a day late arriving at The Olive Press. Still, we do get to experience another olive oil tasting. Olive oil experts will tell you that olive oil must be tasted to be "fully understood and appreciated." Think of wine or coffee aficionados. It takes practice and a knack to be able to differentiate a fine Chardonnay or delicious cup of java.

So, "How will I lose my inhibitions and taste the olive oils at The Olive Press?" I ponder. I rehearse the scenario: Pour a small amount of olive oil into a small cup. (But note, if you are at a tasting bar, this is often already done for you.) Place the cup in the palm of your hand and cover it with your fingers to warm it. After a minute or two, place the cup under your nose to appreciate the aroma of the oil.

I feel too shy to pretend to be Hannibal Lector (from the scene in the film *Silence of the Lambs* where he makes a frightening sucking noise with his mouth) or a veteran judge, so I invite my extroverted friend Jim Berkland, a geologist and longtime resident of Glen Ellen, known for its wineries, to show us the way to The Olive Press and step up to the cup, so to speak. And he did.

It is show time. While I had heard and read about the process, I watch it again take place in front of me. I view Berkland place a small amount of oil on his lower lip and, with the tip of his tongue, taste the oil for its degree of sweetness. Then, using the sides of his tongue, he sips the oil and tastes for spiciness. (I decide I will do the dip-my-bread-into-olive-oil tasting method in the privacy of my own home, in front of my nonjudgmental dogs and cat.)

The last stop is at B.R. Cohn Olive Oil Company in Glen Ellen. Because we are late, our tour has been cancelled. However, I do manage to come home with a Baronessa Cali Oliva Spa Viaggio Travel Set with extracts of Italian olive oil and a bar of Cali olive oil–based soap. And, for some reason, that makes everything all right, because I know I'll be able to pamper myself at home with the natural beauty products from my tour to where olives are blessed once a year.

Note to self: When a snowstorm threatens, go with the flow on an olive oil tasting tour, because you never know what you're going to get. Then again, one olive oil enthusiast got to visit both Napa Valley and Tuscany, and got the best of both worlds. . . .

Olive Alive

The olive trees are here, for sure,
And oh, those trees bring happiness
With olive oil that's mighty pure
For those who find The Olive Press.

The oval leaves of bluish green
Remain alive the whole year long,
And so they grace our country scene,
Although sometimes the trees go wrong.

That's when the ripened olives drop
Unharvested to coat the ground;
And then you may just need a mop,
Or watch your step when you're around.

But olive fruit, when treated right,
Gives salads just a touch of class;
And olives, stuffed, provide delight
When gracing your martini glass.

So olive trees have had their place
In Bible times, as well as now;
They've served to time the human race,
And now 'tis time to take their "bough."
—Jim Berkland
Glen Ellen, California

TUSCANY'S TREES TO NAPA'S OLIVES

Remember the Garden Lady, who gives her dog olive oil in his chow? She and her husband have had the fortunate delight to taste olive oil in Italy and Northern California. When she turned 50 (in 2000), she, C.L. Fornari, and her husband, Dan, went to Tuscany to celebrate. C.L. writes:

Everywhere we went we tasted olive oil. A high point of the trip was walking the Cinque Terre, with olive trees growing on the steep hill to one side and the ocean on the other. We returned with several bottles of olive oil, and since then it has been a tradition to give olive oil as one of our New Year's gifts.

There is no more beautiful and pastoral area than Tuscany. The gently rolling hills display whatever crop is being grown, be it sunflowers or olive trees. The light silver-green color of the olive leaves and the neatly spaced rows of trees that stretch over the hillsides are especially beautiful next to the terra-cotta and burnt sienna colors of the Northern Italian land. One of the many memories that I treasure from this trip is a trip to Venzano, a nursery and garden in Tuscany. En route, we stopped on the side of the road and got out of the car to admire the fields and olive groves. The only sound we heard was the clanking of the distant bells on the sheep in the fields. How rare that is in today's world—to only hear the sound of sheep's bells.

When in Tuscany we were told that the traditional way to test olive oil is to pour some into the palm of your hand and smell it. It should smell fruity and very much of olives. Next, lick it off your palm—the freshest oil will be peppery, and the best will taste as fruity as it smells. In the stores for tourists, they offer small cubes of bread to soak up the oil for tasting, of course, and they often encourage people to start by tasting the blandest oils, working up to the strongest and most spicy. Dan and myself passed the watery oils by and went straight for the strongest stuff: why take in calories with little body and flavor?

Several years later, Dan and C.L. went to the wine country in Northern California. In November, with another couple—both couples celebrating their wedding anniversaries—they stayed at the Beltane Ranch, a historic Sonoma Valley bed and breakfast inn where they grow olives for oil. They tasted olive oils at many places in both Napa and Sonoma counties. Says C.L.:

> We set off in search of Katz and Company winding our way through a fairly industrial section of Napa to what seemed to be an office park. The woman explained that they had closed the Napa tasting room some years ago but she was happy to share their olive oil with us in the middle of the office/storeroom. The owner graciously offered us tastes. We tasted all the "Kitchen Line" offerings, and our favorite by far was the one they called "December Oil"—it is the first, fresh pressing of the season, so it is full of the most peppery olive flavor. That year we ordered "December Oil" Katz and Company for everyone on our New Year's list, and this year I did the same.

The fact remains, there is an art to tasting olive oil, and who better to describe it than an olive oil farmer in Italy. . . .

LIKE AN ITALIAN

"It's up to an official tasters panel to determine the goodness of the oil in a sort of numerical range according to its flavor. But there is nothing to prevent you from personally doing this test much to your delight and satisfaction. Taste is rather subjective," notes olive oil farmer Antonio of Umbria, Italy. Here, take a look at his hands-on olive oil tasting tips:

- The test results will be better if you have not eaten for an hour and not smoked for 30 minutes.
- Take care to cleanse your palate with some water and a piece of bread before each tasting.

- Put a small amount of each of the different oils in different transparent glass bowls to examine their colors.
- Swirl the oil around in the bowl, warming it with your hands (so it can rise above room temperature) and evaluate the oil's fluidity.
- Inhale deeply to note the intensity of the bouquet.
- Take some drops in your mouth and softly put your tongue to your palate to get the first flavors.
- Take a more substantial draught of the oil (a teaspoon), mixing it with air to help release the flavors. Before swallowing, keep it in your mouth for 20 seconds to gradually enjoy the taste.
- Enjoy the intensity of the aftertaste.

I can tell you, though, as an unbiased individual who is a newbie at tasting olive oils, that while experiencing the different olive oils you will wonder, "How can I use this type in my cooking?" According to The Olive Press experts, there are three distinct categories of extra virgin olive oils:

- *Mild:* Buttery, sweet. Perfect with broiled and grilled fish, hot and cold vegetable soups, sauces without garlic, cooked and steamed vegetables, meat and carpaccio, and cheeses.
- *Fruity:* "Olivey," that is, green (tasting of grass, leaves, or fruit) or ripe. Complements grilled meat and vegetables, pasta, bruschetta without garlic, sauces with garlic, and milder cheeses.
- *Fruity-pungent:* Spicy, peppery (perceived in throat). Perfectly complements traditional, rustic dishes such as bruschetta with garlic, pasta e fagioli (pasta and beans), ribollita (vegetable-and-bread soup), and panzella (tomato-and-bread salad).

AN OLIVE OIL TOUR DE FORCE

While going to Umbria to taste olive oil is my dream, it isn't necessary to fly thousands of miles to do so. But some people in the world will trek far enough to get the good stuff. Sara Conley, an olive oil enthusiast, recalls an exciting adventure that she shared with her boyfriend, Robert A. Salitore II. She told me, "We flew from O'Hare International to San Luis Obispo County airport via L.A. on Thursday, November 30. We were lucky enough to stay in the little white cottage on the ranch as guests. Rob and I weren't afraid to try the oil right after pressing because the Pasolivo oil is so flavorful to begin with, and we are such huge fans, we knew it would be right up our alley."

Rob vividly recollects the unforgettable olive oil touring adventure at Paso Robles, California, on December 1, 2006. . . .

On this day a group of us who love the peppery, green goodness of Pasolivo are assembled to see how it all happens. Dressed in boots and work clothes, we've come to see the oil made from start to finish.

Joeli Yaguda leads us out into the olive orchard. We get the history of the ranch on the way over and her love for the place shines through. Then, we arrive at our row of trees, with their silvery green leaves and limbs drooping with ripe olives. Each of the 17 of us either straps a bucket to the front of our chest or carries one by hand. We are shown by the ranch manager how to glide one hand down the limb and direct the olives into the bucket. He gets every olive off in one clean motion. He's a pro.

Then, we're off into the trees. We have to keep to the low hangers because no ladders are allowed. We strip olives from the tree with both hands while hearing the thump, thump, thump as they hit the bottom of the bucket. We're told to pick all of the olives, green and black alike. It seems when you harvest an olive tree you harvest them all, ripe or not so ripe.

Everyone in the group is getting into the process and after an hour we picked 308 pounds. We beat the group who had visited the day before and a group of 2nd graders from the previous week. We've all warmed up substantially, taken off our outer layers, and gaze at our collection as workers all around us continue climbing trees and harvesting. They've been there since 5 A.M. and will continue working into the night. The entire harvest takes two weeks of 12 hour days and we were lucky enough to experience it.

Back at the tasting room and mill we sit down for a sensory analysis. We are each served three olive oils blindly. We pick up the glass to warm it, then lift our hand to let the aroma surround our nose. We take in the fruity, grass smell and then lift the glass, one by one, to our lips. Amazing.

Back out in the mill room, the olives we've harvested are getting a bath. Afterward they ride up a conveyor and inside to the mill, which whirrs and whirrs without stopping. Soon I'm brought over to a barrel which is being fed a stream of neon green liquid from an overhead pipe. This is olive oil made from olives that I harvested with my own hands hours before. I'm given a small pitcher which I dip under the liquid. I insert a funnel into a small bottle and pour from the pitcher the freshest olive oil I could ever imagine. Next comes a stopper and a label, and we're in business. I feel so connected to the oil, and wish I had a hand in making all of the food and wine I consume. Modern life really doesn't afford us that opportunity, but I am grateful for the chance to go from olive to oil with my very own hands.

As you can see, olive oil producers, tasting bars, and tours can be found in Northern and Southern California as well as in Italy—the place I plan to go one day, especially now that I am learning to appreciate olives and olive oil.

In fact, Gloria Cappelli and her partner, Marcel C. Gordon, described to me their vacation rental. Here, let her paint the postcard-perfect picture for you if you're looking for a holiday home in Tuscany. . . .

Casina di Rosa is an old 19th century village house; my great-grandparents built it over 100 years ago. It never left the family, and in 2003 when we had to face the choice of selling or doing something with it, since it had been empty for quite a while, we decided to try and rent it by the week to foreign guests. I am from the village, Civtella Marittima. Both my parents were also from the village. I am very fond of the area, which is called Upper Maremma and is part of Tuscany. The house is very tiny, only 400 square feet. There are four rooms: a kitchen with the old fireplace which we kept in the renovation, the bedroom, a sitting room which we have equipped with guidebooks and books about olive oil, the bathroom. By the main entrance there is a small patio with two chairs to enjoy the morning sun and watch the village life go by.

Siena is one of the most beautiful cities in Tuscany. Grosseto is the capital of the Maremma, a subregion of Tuscany, scarcely populated by Italian standards. The house is in the village, so there are other stone houses, little streets, and great views over the valley, as the village is on the top of a hill. Just walk five minutes and you will find as many olive trees as you wish.

My father has olive groves all around the village. When I am available I take guests to our fields, otherwise Carlo Barbieri takes them to Podere Vignali where it is like *Under the Tuscan Sun*, maybe better. In small villages, reaching the farmed countryside is so easy that it is like living in the countryside itself.

For more information, log onto http://www.casinadirosa.it/.

A DAY IN A LIFE WITH OLIVE OIL

Whether you live in Chicago, Tuscany, or Lake Tahoe, olive oil—and its products—can lure you to travel to see what the olive oil world is all about. Take a look at my new daily agenda, which revolves around the healing powers of oil. In the cold, dry mountain winter climate of Lake Tahoe, I don't know how I survived without it.

8:00 A.M.: Spray the frying pan with extra virgin olive oil before I scramble two eggs. Gemma Sciabica taught me this trick, and it works like a charm. No more brown, toasty eggs on my plate.

8:30 A.M.: Shower with olive oil–based soap (rosemary/sage); wash hair with olive oil–based shampoo and crème rinse.

8:45 A.M.: Massage extra virgin olive oil into my feet and hands.

9:00 A.M.: Too cold to shampoo the dogs, so I put a drop of extra virgin olive oil on Simon's back and brush him thoroughly. Ditto for Seth.

10:00 A.M.: Water houseplants in the dining room and spritz with a mixture of water and olive oil.

Noon: Warm up French bread in the microwave along with a small bowl of flavored olive oil. Toss together a salad of greens, tuna, tomatoes, olive oil, and red wine vinegar.

1:00 P.M.: Use olive oil and lemon to dust the desk and living room table in an attempt to remove teacup rings.

5:00 P.M.: Order a vegetarian pizza: spinach, tomatoes, mushrooms, and olives.

5:30 P.M.: Bring in wood for the fire. Wash my hands and rub olive oil moisturizing hand lotion on my cuticles after making the fire.

9:00 P.M.: Give myself a pedicure. After the polish has dried, I apply olive oil generously to the bottoms of my feet and put on fresh socks for the rest of the evening.

10:00 P.M.: Wipe out both Brittanys' ear canals with extra virgin olive oil. They're going to the vet tomorrow, and I want them to be clean for the technician.

11:00 P.M.: Take a primose oil gelcap and hope that it will help deal with post-menopausal woes.

Midnight: Take a quick glance at *The Healing Powers of Olive Oil,* the new edition, to make sure I've added new ways I can use versatile, all-natural olive oil (and other oils) to make my life easier and more bearable in the mountains.

Now that you know everything good you wanted to know about olive oil but were afraid to ask, let's take a close-up and personal look at the downside (unfortunately, not even olive oil is 100 percent perfect) of this healing liquid.

Crostini with Basil, Garlic, Goat Cheese, and Sun-Dried Tomato Topping

❖ ❖ ❖

The best way to make bread for crostini is in French baguette pans. The resulting loaves, long and skinny, make bite-sized crostini when sliced into thin rounds, ideal for appetizers. Simply grease the pans and scoop the dough into them, stretching and patting it to fit with lightly greased fingers. There's no need to try to roll the dough into a log and transfer it to the pan; though the stretching and patting method makes a messy-looking loaf at first, once it's risen and baked, it will be as smooth as any shaped loaf.

CROSTINI LOAVES

2 teaspoons instant yeast
1½ teaspoons salt
2 teaspoons granulated
    sugar
Coarse semolina or corn-
    meal for the pan

3 cups (12¾ ounces)
    unbleached all purpose
    flour
¼ cup (1¾ ounces) olive oil

TOPPING

16 ounces goat cheese
    (plain or herbed)
1 to 1½ heads fresh garlic,
    cloves separated, peeled,
    and sliced thin
Coarse semolina or corn-
    meal for the pan

3 cups loosely packed fresh
    basil leaves
2 to 3 cups (9 to 14 ounces)
    sun-dried tomato slices
    packed in oil, drained
    (snipped in half if large)

TO MAKE THE LOAVES

In the bowl of an electric mixer or the bucket of a bread machine, combine all the ingredients, mixing until a rough dough forms. If using a mixer, knead dough with the flat beater for about 7 minutes; it will become smooth but won't form a ball or clean the sides of the bowl. Transfer the dough to a lightly greased bowl, cover the bowl with lightly greased plastic wrap, and let the dough rise for 1 hour.

Transfer the dough to a lightly oiled work surface. Divide it into three pieces. If you're using a baguette pan, grease the molds of the pan and sprinkle them with coarse semolina or yellow cornmeal. Working with one piece at a time, lay the dough in the pan and stretch and pat it to within 1 inch of each end. Repeat with the remaining pieces of dough. If you're not using a baguette pan, pat the dough as best you can into three 16-inch logs and place them on two lightly oiled baking sheets. Cover the dough with lightly oiled plastic wrap or a proof cover and set aside to rise until it's very puffy, 1 to 1½ hours.

When the bread has risen, preheat the oven to 425°.

Bake the loaves for 20 to 25 minutes, until they're golden brown. Remove the loaves from the oven and transfer them to a wire rack to cool completely. When the bread is cool, drape it with a cloth towel and let it rest overnight; it needs to be a bit stale before you cut it.

Preheat the oven to 275°. Slice the bread crosswise into ½-inch rounds. Pour a generous coating of olive oil (about ⅛ inch) into a couple of half-sheet pans or two large cookie sheets with sides; use your fingers to spread the oil completely over the bottom of the pans. Put the bread slices in the pans in one layer, as close together as you can get them. Drizzle the slices lightly with olive oil (or spray them with olive oil spray) and bake them for 45 minutes, or until they're very dry and are just beginning to brown. Remove the crostini from the oven and let them cool.

If not serving them the same day, store the crostini in an airtight container.

To Make the Topping

Note that all of the amounts are approximate. You'll use more or less depending on a variety of factors, including the size of the basil leaves and tomatoes, how thin you slice the garlic, and how generous you are with the cheese. To say nothing of how many crostini you've sampled before even getting to the topping. If you find yourself with leftover topping ingredients, make a salad.

Gently crumble the goat cheese into a small bowl. Spread each crostini with 1 teaspoon of cheese, then top with a basil leaf, a slice or slices of garlic, and a sun-dried tomato slice, snipped in half if overly large. Serve immediately; the crostini will get soggy if they wait more than about half an hour. Serve as an appetizer or as part of a large antipasto. Makes about 9 dozen.

(Courtesy: The King Arthur Flour Baker's Companion: The All-Purpose Baking Cookbook)

THE GOLDEN SECRETS TO REMEMBER

✓ Harvest season is from fall to late winter, and olive oil can vary in taste depending on the time of year it is made.

✓ Spain, Italy, and Greece are the regions where olive oil production is most prevalent, but olive oil producers exist around the globe.

✓ People use a variety of terms, such as "bitter" and "flat," when judging the flavor of an olive oil.

✓ Northern California is gaining in popularity as a place where award-winning olive oils are produced; tours and tasting bars are very vogue.

✓ Olive oil enthusiasts, much like wine lovers, will travel to Tuscany and Northern California to tour, taste, and bring home artisanal olive oils.

✓ While the Golden State's olives are grown in Northern California, central California also has its place in the olive oil world.

✓ In the twenty-first century, you don't have to travel anywhere to indulge in olive oil and its array of products. Olive oil is everywhere, and you can use it for cooking, bathing, cleaning, beauty, pet care, and so much more, just like in ancient biblical times.

Olive Oil Is Not for Everyone: Some Bitter Views

England and the English, as a rule they will refuse even to sample a foreign dish, they regard such things as garlic and olive oil with disgust, life is unliveable to them unless they have tea and puddings.

—George Orwell[1]

When working on this book, I opened the kitchen pantry a lot, and sometimes I'd get flashbacks of my youthful twenties, the time when I didn't cook and bake as much as I wanted to do it. I was without a kitchen to call my own. In Southern California, my Golden State, to Eugene, Oregon, I was a changing hippie girl (like an olive tree) couch-surfing amid friends with dreams of establishing roots in the future.

On a cold and cloudy Christmas Day, a group of us young nomads drove out to Newport, to a friend's beach home. A woman in her thirties made a large dinner, complete with ham, potatoes, pies, and cookies. We were invited to indulge in the meal. I recall there were no oils and no butter. Instead, margarine and store-bought salad dressings in bottles were passed around the table. It wasn't an unforgettable pesto pasta night like my godmother had made or the Thanksgiving dinner with flavored oils and flavorful food on the coast in Santa Cruz.

The dinner was bland, but the surroundings were amazing. In the bathroom with amazing décor—from a claw bathtub to seashell shower curtain—I fantasized about having my own kitchen. I envisioned me cooking and baking all day. I made a vow that day. I'd be in my own house with a fireplace, nestled amid towering trees, a dog, and cooking with herbs, spices, and nature's oils and fats. But I never dreamed I, the picky eater, would be sharing my down-to-earth recipes with readers.

Speaking of olive oil aficionados, there are some people who cannot and will not tolerate the golden liquid. While olive oil can be used both inside and outside the body, some people insist it causes problems.

Taking a tablespoon or two of olive oil solo on a daily basis (like Professor Seth Roberts did to maintain his weight loss) may not be the perfect remedy for everyone. There are people who have turned to olive oil for good health and other uses, but there are many others who have made an oil change or are turned off by olive oil for different reasons. Here's why.

TOO MUCH OF A GOOD THING

Does all this good news about olive oil nudge you to run, not walk, to your nearest supermarket, health food store, or online retailer for a bottle of the golden liquid? If so, remember that olive oil and other oils are not calorie-free. One tablespoon of the elixir with healing powers boasts 120 calories, give or take a few. That means, calorie-wise, you can't pour the golden liquid on everything from pasta and potatoes to dipping bread and bagels. Doing so can cause a good thing to have weighty results. Translation: It isn't difficult to pack on unwanted pounds fast if you overdo it with olive oil, or with any food that packs calories—"good" fat or not. But even if you don't go overboard, you may run into another problem.

SENSITIVITY TO OLIVE OIL

One woman, for example, claims her boyfriend, a no-nonsense globetrotter, enjoys olive oil–based recipes in his travels to places like Greece and Spain. Unfortunately, within 30 minutes, the adventurous foodie ends up in the restroom for longer than he'd prefer.

According to John Deane, M.D., "Sensitivity to olive oil is rare but certainly possible. If the oil cannot be absorbed for some reason, it will act as a cathartic. Extra virgin olive oil is not processed, the olives are simply ground up and the oil removed by pressing or spinning in a centrifuge."

He adds, "The type of olives used for oil production may contain as much as 20% of their weight in oil. The larger varieties grown for pickling and brining often have as little as 5% oil, so it is not surprising that eating olives doesn't cause the same problem."

BAKING BLUNDERS

Gemma Sciabica, a nutrition-savvy woman and, as I've noted, the author of five cookbooks, guarantees that olive oil can and does work in baking, even in double-layer chocolate cakes and pie crusts for your favorite apples. Note to self: I will try both.

But, some folks don't have pleasant experiences with olive oil in their baking adventures. A Midwest writer, for one, explains that she loves olive oil. "However, olive oil only goes so far. For my birthday, my husband made me a dark chocolate cake and, not being a baker, he didn't even notice the difference between the two oils (canola and olive) and the cake was unbearable; although it was moist, it had this thick, distinct olive oily taste that overpowered the dark chocolate. But I was just so happy for the effort I barely noticed. The next day, the cake found its way to the Dumpster."

Another fellow writer recalls, "The only olive oil story I have is that it put me in the doghouse. My girlfriend was making last-minute pumpkin bread for a party and got mad at me when I tried to use olive oil in place of vegetable oil. (I told her we had oil when she was out shopping.)"

So, what was the end result? "My girlfriend wouldn't let me use the olive oil and sent the first person to arrive at our party to the store to buy canola oil. Funny, she usually enjoys olive oil, but for some reason felt this olive oil discrimination and guest imposition was worth it. The pumpkin bread has so much sugar in it that I'm pretty sure Brylcreem would have worked in place of the oil," adds the disgruntled boyfriend, who believes olive oil would have sufficed. And that's not all . . .

CAN OLIVE OIL GO BAD?

Since I'm on a roll regarding worst-case-scenario olive oil stories, I might as well include my own personal experience. Blame it on my lack of knowledge about cooking and storing cooking oils. In my thirties, a friend of mine was moving to Los Angeles. In return, I got to stock my pantry with lots of his kitchen cupboard goodies—including a bottle of olive oil.

One night, I got the desire to whip up a pasta dish. I used all fresh vegetables and pasta. Then, I tossed it with the olive oil. (Remember, I knew nothing at all about the shelf life of oils.) So, I didn't think twice about its longevity, assuming it was like a good wine, which gets better as it ages, right? One hour later: I was dead wrong. In the bathroom, I grew very sick. The bottom line: The olive oil was rancid, and I will never forget it. I tossed it for good.

So, how long does olive oil last, anyhow? You'll find different answers to this question. It isn't cut-and-dried as for vinegar, which does get better with age.The consensus is, store it in a cool, dark place. Also, keep it away from heat. But note: Some types of oils, such as flavored oils, nut, and seed oils, should be refrigerated.

The shelf life of an olive oil product depends on a variety of things, such as storage time, temperature, age, and container. I suggest you contact the manufacturer if you have any concerns rather than pull a stunt like I did and end up in the bathroom wishing you had the right knowledge about the shelf life of olive oil. I prefere using olive oil products that include an expiration date.

FAKE OLIVE OIL: ARE YOU SURE THAT'S REAL?

While olive oil can go rancid, it also can be an imposter. Welcome to the world of fake foods. Did you know that some food manufacturers, big and small around the globe, sneak cheaper ingredients into their products that you eat? Yes, it's true that what you're eating may not be true. The thing is, certain foods are pricey to produce and make a profit. So switching the fake stuff for the real deal is a ploy fooling folks like you and me. Here, take an up-close and very unsettling peek at some common fake eats—the earthy news may open your eyes to reality bites no matter where you live.

IS IT REALLY VIRGIN OLIVE OIL?

People in the olive oil world, including the North American Olive Oil Association, know that the olive oil in some grocery stores and dollar stores may not be 100 percent pure, but instead be "adulterated" (contaminated with tainted elements). And these oils can come from Asia all the way to the United States.

This fact is upsetting to people because we are not only not getting what we pay for, but we also are being duped. Often the olive oil is watered down with other oils, like canola, sunflower, or cheaper oils. This ordeal has made headlines in the news such as "Is Your Olive Oil Fake?" and "The Great Olive Oil Fraud," and it's causing concern for both consumers and olive oil producers.

Like chocolate, olive oil can be heart healthy, and it's a fact that extra virgin olive oil (EVOO) with Italian roots is the preferred grade. Extra virgin means the olive oil is extracted from the highest quality olives. It must have less than 1 percent natural acidity. Its fruity flavor is intense.

Fresh-pressed extra virgin olive oil can be enjoyed without chemical processing. Olive oil gurus will tell you that it retains the natural flavors, vitamins, minerals, antioxidants, and other healthy products of the ripe olive fruit. But the glitch is, some manufacturers, not unlike in the honey and chocolate worlds, are fudging and labeling their oil as "extra virgin" when it's not pure. So are you purchasing and consuming fake olive oil? It is sold as extra virgin olive oil in Italy and the Americas. But raids to arrests and tests allow oils to be certified pure "extra virgin olive oil"—yet countless imported brands of EVOO have flunked the test.

I went straight to the North American Olive Oil Association to get the scoop on olive oil. "Most claims of 'fake' olive oil are based on hearsay," said Eryn Balch, vice president of the NAOOA. While the University of California Davis research provides claims of fraud with percentages (that are perhaps a bit biased), the NAOOA quality seal program does its own tests. The association pulls brands from retail shelves and food service distributors at least twice a year, I'm told. Its mission is to test extra virgin olive oil with certified International Olive Council (IOC) labs and panels. And there's more.

History tells us that the NAOOA has been collecting about 150–200 samples of olive oil from all over the nation each year for more than two decades. We're talking samples and more samples of olive oil that are tested with "a full battery of chemical analysis to check for compliance with the IOC grade standards for olive oil," explained Balch. The end results: Approximately eight percent may have issues, but the problems, according to the NAOOA, are a small percentage. So while headlines pop up in the media from time to time, the key is to understand that olive oil goes bad—especially with handling and storage. Check your expiration labels, too. But it doesn't stop there.

OTHER HEALING FOODS ARE NOT IMMUNE

- Imitation honeys are not a sweet matter in the real world. That means trouble lies ahead for real honey lovers who want to "save the endangered honey bear." Honey-flavored syrups, or honey that's diluted with other ingredients, are becoming more commonplace and being sold to the unaware consumer. To be sure you get the pure golden food of the gods, check the label and source of honey. All-natural, 100 percent pure honey will have the ingredients listed on the nutrition label: honey.

- Quality imitation dark chocolate, much like imitation honeys, can haunt chocolate lovers, too. While we're talking good and bad honey, in the United States some chocolate manufacturers began to use less expensive hydrogenated vegetable oil in the place of cocoa butter to be sold as "chocolate" (which was reported by the news several years ago). Consumers won the battle of "Is it real or fake chocolate?" thanks to the FDA, and labeling will now note whether chocolate contains vegetable oil or the real stuff—cocoa butter. This is important because cocoa butter contains oleic acid (a heart-healthy monounsaturated fat). So if this good fat goes AWOL, health-conscious, no-nonsense chocolate fans won't be smiling or buying the fake food from the gods.

- Just when you think you paid the price for in-demand, delicious Hawaiian "Kona" java beans, you may be one of countless coffee drinkers not getting "Kona blend coffee"—the words stamped on labels of coffee bags for sale and profit. Evidently, the truth was stretched too far. The sobering news is, the coffee didn't make the grade at Safeway Inc., which reached a 2013 class action lawsuit settlement with consumers who weren't smiling with the grocery chain committing fraud by pushing coffee tagged as a Kona blend even though it contained only a small proportion of Kona beans.

Meanwhile, you can play a food sleuth and weed out fake foods including olive oil and other superfoods. And note, it's in your best interest to get olive oil, chocolate, coffee, and honey from reputable producers and/or locally to help ensure you're getting the real stuff, and that'll provide peace of mind for your body and spirit.

HARD TO SWALLOW

Statistics continue to show that olive oil is growing in popularity because of its healing perks. But that doesn't mean everyone can take a tablespoon (or two) per day like Dr. Seth Roberts to maintain his or her weight, dip his or her bread into the warm oil, or drizzle it on his or her salad. So, what do you do if you want the health benefits but can't bear to swallow this important food?

Olive leaf extract may be the answer for you. Yes, you can get condensed olive oil in tea, capsules, and other forms, and it may be easier for you to take. There are many health food stores that carry a variety of olive leaf extract products.

As time goes on, my prediction in the first edition that olive oil—and other healing oils—will be used in more kitchens around the globe is coming true. Not only is it part of a healthful Mediterranean diet (which is being put to work more and more for good health), but it has earned its good household name. Last and by no means least, in Chapter 18, "The Joy of Cooking with Olive Oil," I am pleased to share creative and nutritious cooking tips.

Banana Nutty Muffins

❖ ❖ ❖

On one Sunday afternoon, I baked banana muffins in my Old Tahoe kitchen with its rustic Mediterranean décor and colors. I turned on the oven and went to work like a worker bee. With a backdrop of a wood-paneled wall lined with bookshelves high with my published books (in different languages) and articles—it made me recall how I've made the gift of banana nut bread during both my best and worst of times, with tribute to Charles Dickens. This is one of my own recipes that you can make for friends and family who claim they don't like the taste of olive oil but will unwittingly get the gift of gold.

½ cup organic brown sugar
2 tablespoons extra virgin olive oil
1 tablespoon each macadamia nut oil, walnut oil, and European-style butter
2 brown eggs
¼ cup low-fat buttermilk
2 ripe organic bananas, mashed

2 cups whole wheat flour
½ teaspoon baking soda
1½ teaspoons baking powder
2 tablespoons orange blossom honey
½ teaspoon vanilla
1 teaspoon allspice
½ cup walnuts, chopped
Raw cane sugar (for sprinkling)

Cream together sugar, oils, and butter in a bowl; add eggs, buttermilk and bananas. Combine dry ingredients: flour, soda, and baking powder. Add honey, vanilla, allspice, and walnuts. Pour into two lightly buttered or olive-oil-greased bread loaf pans. Bake at 350° for about 30–40 minutes until firm and golden brown. Sprinkle sugar on top. Cool. Makes 12 muffins.

THE GOLDEN SECRETS TO REMEMBER

- ✓ Olive oil can be one person's best medicine and another individual's worst nightmare, depending on how it's used and the person who uses it.
- ✓ A sensitivity to olive oil—like a sensitivity to anything—can happen, but it isn't common.
- ✓ Pay attention to the "use by" date. You do not want to use olive oil that has expired.
- ✓ Olive oil and other oils can and are used in baking every day, and have been for years.
- ✓ Keep in mind that food chains across the nation—starting in New York—are banning unhealthy trans fats from muffins, cookies, and other baked goods, and replacing them with healthier oils.

The Joy of Cooking
with Olive Oil

EVOO.
—Rachael Ray

My fantasy of cooking and baking dishes in my own dwelling didn't become a reality for years. During a past Thanksgiving holiday in the Sierra, I was preparing game (only on special occasions or when I dabble with the Paleo diet to lose a few unwanted pounds) glazed with honey vinegar and sweet potato pie with an olive oil crust. I was haunted by a meal of the past that made me feel like a chef getting chopped on a TV show on the Food Network.

I was invited to an ex-boyfriend's mother's home for Christmas dinner. Jackie lived to eat while I ate to live. I put together a modest meal due to budget constraints. And, I admit, my lack of culinary skills left my entrée and dessert nondescript. My tree was crooked like a sad and small Charlie Brown attempt; the lights were mismatched, ornaments not all silver, gold, and red like her tree of perfection. My ineptitude in the kitchen and holiday decorations would have made any celeb chef judge bring me to tears.

Upon arriving at Ms. Martha Stewart's understudy, I felt at ease sitting on her patio surrounded by Boston ferns in the winter sunshine. The Christmas tree was tall with dozens of stuffed brown bears dressed with red and black, plaid ribbon bowties. The table spread looked like a gourmet food magazine layout. I felt like a culinary failure (or as if I were an olive tree not adequate during harvest time). As I nibbled on each dish, I secretly was plotting a redo that didn't make me feel like a failure, but a real chef who gets foods and flavors. But that day didn't arrive anytime soon. Enter olive oil. . . .

World-renowned chef Mario Batali has said that "olive oil is as precious as gold." Television personality Rachael Ray, a Food Network regular, uses catchy phrases such as "EVOO" in reference to extra virgin olive oil. What's more, the word is that Ray's acronym, EVOO, is being added to the Oxford American College Dictionary.

It's no secret that chefs, on the little and big screens, in restaurants and their own kitchens, treasure olive oil, be it on the West Coast, East Coast, or Mediterranean basin.

The recipes in *The Healing Powers of Olive Oil* are created with fresh superfoods—nutrient-dense vegetables, fruits, grains, legumes, fish, poultry, and olive oil. Our wide array of dishes, provided by chefs from Europe and olive oil experts who have visited Spain, Italy, and Greece, contain a variety of oils—olive oil, flaxseed oil, canola oil, and herbal oils. Plus, good-for-you garlic, onions, and red wine and balsamic vinegars are often part of the recipes, too.

For best results, use the olive oil brand noted in each recipe. However, feel free to use your own brand or a brand without sodium (you want to keep unwanted pounds and high blood pressure at bay, whatever age you are). Or, if you are lean and have normal blood pressure, treat yourself to the wide collection of specialty flavored olive oils.

Before you begin, take a look at some tips for cooking with olive oil, which can help you make these recipes turn out fabulous. Olive oil and other oils teamed with health-boosting, good-for-you foods will not only keep your weight in check but may add years to your life. It was my intention to bring European flair to your kitchen, since not all of us can whisk away to Italy in a heartbeat. So, use a variety of these original, healthful, and delicious recipes perfect for a heart-healthy, anti-cancer, Mediterranean-style diet. If you're like me (an accidental health-conscious foodie), or if you are an adventurous foodie, you may wonder what took you so long to cook up an olive oil-based delight paired with healthful companion foods. It's a healthy romance with food that I, and you, can savor time after time year round.

THE WORLD OF OILS

So, what oils should you use in cooking? Roe Valenti, a veteran chef and caterer who cooks for herself, her family, and her friends, told me she likes to cook with only one oil—olive oil. When I asked her, "Why olive oil?" she had the answer.

"When I was a kid, my grandmother used to tell me, 'Don't ever use anything other than olive oil. It's good for you.' So olive oil was part of my daily diet. You know us Italians. We use olive oil for everything, from salads to pasta. Perhaps that's why our record for longevity is a good one."[1]

The only other oil she recommended is canola, to make your own salad dressing or to put in your water when you're going to boil pasta. "Aside from these uses, it's olive oil all the way. And it's funny, because when I go to a friend's house to make dinner they know they will get a healthy meal. But, when I say, 'I'm going to sauté the veggies first' the response is the same, 'You're going to sauté the food with oil?' I answer, 'Yes, with olive oil, there is no need to worry.' Then, after I get the taste from the olive oil combined into the food I'm cooking, that's it. Any other moisture I get is from wine, broth or water."[2]

Italians like Valenti love olive oil—but there are so many types of oil, as you know—including the wide world of flavored oils. Take a look and see how you can put to use the wonderful flavors of olive oil in your cooking.

OILS WITH HEART AND SOUL!

Oil	Flavor	Uses
Canola oil	Mild	All purpose for cooking, salads, baking
Extra virgin olive oil	Fruity, intense	Drizzling, salads, marinades, sauces, stews, soups
Virgin olive oil	Strong, but milder than EVOO	Grilling, sautéing, drizzling, salad dressings, marinades, stews, soups
Peanut oil	Intense	Stir-fries, sautéing
Olive oil	Mild	Baking, frying, grilling, sautéing
Light olive oil	Very mild	Baking, frying, grilling, sautéing

OILS WITH HEART AND SOUL! (*cont.*)

Oil	Flavor	Uses
Basil olive oil	Fresh taste in pesto	Dipping, drizzling, vegetables, tomatoes, tomato-based sauces, Southeast Asian cuisine, soups, salads, pastas, stir-fries
Garlic-flavored olive oil	Zesty, added zip	Sautéing, vegetables, pasta
Jalapeño olive oil	Hot, peppery	Southwest dishes, eggs
Lemon-flavored olive oil	Tangy, light	Salads, fish, chicken
Lime-flavored olive oil	Tangy, light	Salads, fish
Orange-flavored olive oil	Tangy, light	Chicken, duck
Oregano olive oil	Intense	Tomatoes, pizza, tomato-based sauces, pasta, dressings
Pepper olive oil	Hot, peppery	Sautéing, roasting, eggs, seafood, Southwest cuisine

OILS WITH HEART AND SOUL! (*cont.*)

Oil	Flavor	Uses
Porcini olive oil	Sweet	Vegetable dishes
Rosemary olive oil	Strong, pungent	Roasted potatoes, eggplant, artichokes, asparagus, dressings, breads
Tangerine olive oil	Tangy, light	Salads, chicken

On Top of Old Smoky Point of Oils

Here are some of my favorite cooking oils and their smoke points (there are too many to list all oils and fats).

Oil Type	Smoke–Point Temperature
Almond	430°
Avocado	485°
Canola	400°
Coconut	350°
Extra virgin olive	420°
Flaxseed	225°
Grapeseed	485°

Oil Type	Smoke–Point Temperature
Hemp	330°
Macadamia	389°
Peanut	440°
Red palm	437°
Rice bran	450°
Safflower	320°
Sesame	410°
Soy	350°
Walnut	400°

ROME IN A BOTTLE

Speaking of storing olive oil, C. L. Fornari, aka "The Garden Lady," who has experienced tasting tours in Tuscany and gives her pooch olive oil, has more to say about how she preserves her olive oil in her kitchen. . . .

I keep the following objects right next to my stove: a jar of spatulas, strainers and wooden spoons, another filled only with pairs of scissors, and a third filled with potholders. In front of these are salt and pepper grinders and a dark green glass bottle of olive oil. I consider olive oil to be more important than the salt and pepper, and since I usually leave salt out of recipes and often leave the addition of pepper for when the dish hits the table, the olive oil is probably the most important ingredient on my kitchen counter.

I use a dark green bottle here because the light breaks down the oil when it's in a clear glass container. I have a fancy olive oil bottle with a nicely designed metal pouring spout, but the glass is clear so I seldom use it. I'll purchase one of the less expensive oils in a dark green bottle, or refill an empty bottle from a can of oil that is kept in my cool garage.

Ah, that reminds me: My husband's family are Italian Jews, from Rome. During the second World War Dan's father enlisted in the U.S. Army and worked in Army Counter Intelligence because he spoke several languages, but his mother's family went into hiding in the Italian countryside south of Rome. They were lucky enough to have land where they could raise their own food, as well as grapes and olives that could be traded for other things. After the war Dan's mother and father (not married during the war, but they were high school sweethearts) met up again and got married, and came to this country in the late 1940s. The land where his mother's family was in hiding is now in other hands, but continues to produce olive oil and wine. A cousin orders several large cans of oil from the owners each year and sells them to whomever is interested. Feeling a connection to that place and the olive trees on the farm, we always buy some.

LEARNING TO LOVE OLIVE OIL

I have read how olive oil lovers swear off butter and embrace olive oil as their fat of choice. I admit, it takes a while to get used to the change, just like when you switch to drinking tea instead of soda or eating dark chocolate instead of milk chocolate. But if you do it for 30 days, people say it will become habit. Also, combining a dab of butter or pairing olive oil with another healing oil can give you the best benefits of both oils and fats.

If you love chocolate, you can learn to love olive oil and get a double heart-healthy fix. Recently, I baked brownies. Okay, I didn't make them from scratch, but I did include three eggs (the kind with omega-3s), dark chocolate, fresh walnuts, whole wheat flour (I live in a high altitude), and extra virgin olive oil. Yes, they were tasty and, most likely, healthier than packaged brownies. Next, I will bake a cake with olive oil—such as The Olive Press Citrus Cake (and top it with fresh berries). It is included in the following five-day menu plan.

THE OLIVE OIL HEALTH-BOOSTING FIVE-DAY MENU PLAN

This five-day "California Olive Oil Diet" is based on a nutritious and slimming diet plan I created years ago. It is the way I eat now, too. But I have enhanced it with heart-healthy, irresistible Mediterranean dishes. (Asterisks indicate recipes in Part 7, "Olive Oil Recipes.")

Day 1

Breakfast:
   1 serving oatmeal with low-fat milk and 1 tablespoon raisins

1 orange
Apple Nut Morning Muffin*
1 boiled egg

Lunch:

1 cup non-fat or low-fat yogurt
½ cup raw baby carrots with Golden State Olive Dip
   (Mix together ⅔ cup plain low-fat yogurt, ¼ cup
   finely minced red onion, 2 tablespoons sliced olives,
   1 tablespoon minced fresh chives, and 1 tablespoon
   chopped fresh garlic.)
Caesar Salad*
1 plain whole wheat bagel

Snack:

Fresh fruit
Herbal tea

Dinner:

Simple Salmon*
1 baked potato drizzled with flavored olive oil and diced
   tomatoes
1 slice French bread dipped in olive oil
1 glass red wine or herbal tea

Snack:

Fresh fruit

Day 2

Breakfast:

1 serving whole grain cereal
1 cup skim or low-fat milk
6 ounces fresh carrot or papaya juice

Lunch:
    Cioppino*
    1 cup leafy spinach with red wine vinegar and olive oil
        dressing
    1 slice French bread dipped in olive oil
    1 cup non-fat or low-fat yogurt

Snack:
    Fresh fruit

Dinner:
    Cioppino*
    1 cup fresh fruit salad

Snack:
    1 slice The Olive Press Citrus Cake*

Day 3

Breakfast:
    2 eggs, scrambled in frying pan lightly sprayed with
        olive oil
    Orange Olive Bread*
    6 ounces fresh juice

Lunch:
    3 ounces tuna and ½ cup leafy spinach stuffed into a
        whole wheat pita pocket with ½ sliced tomato and
        alfalfa sprouts
    8 ounces skim or low-fat milk

Snack:
    Fresh fruit

Dinner:

Stir-Fry Shrimp Linguini*
Tossed green salad with vinegar dressing
1 cup broccoli or asparagus spears

Snack:

Fresh fruit

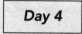

Day 4

Breakfast:

½ cup low-fat granola
½ cup skim milk
1 orange
Whole grain toast with honey

Lunch:

Open-faced grilled cheese sandwich with avocado and
    tomato slices
1 cup gazpacho soup
1 cup fresh fruit salad

Snack:

Rocky Road Tea Bark*

Dinner:

Herbed Roast Turkey*
½ cup mashed potatoes
½ cup green vegetable drizzled with lemon olive oil

Snack:

½ cup vanilla ice cream drizzled with balsamic vinegar

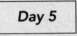

Breakfast:
Vegetable omelet (Sauté ¼ cup each broccoli, red onion, and red bell pepper in 1 teaspoon olive oil for 5–10 minutes. Whisk together 1 egg and 2 egg whites and pour over vegetables. Sprinkle with Cheddar cheese before serving.)
½ cup skim or low-fat milk
6 ounces fresh juice

Lunch:
1 tomato slice and skim Mozzarella cheese grilled on whole grain bagel half and drizzled with olive oil
1 apple
1 cup skim or low-fat milk

Snack:
Fresh olives with Golden State Olive Dip (See Day 1 lunch for recipe.)

Dinner:
Halibut with Caper Sauce*
Garden Salad with Vinaigrette*
1 slice French bread drizzled with olive oil

Snack:
Fresh fruit

Now that you've learned everything you wanted to know about olive oil but were afraid to ask, it's time to bring in recipes for your olive oil future, in Part 7, "Olive Oil Recipes."

Minted Citrus Tea Cookies

❖ ❖ ❖

Later, I will give you my own recipes to use for each season—winter, spring, summer, and fall. You will see that using seasonal foods enhances nature and wholesome eating. Using a variety of olive oils and other healing oils (and fats) also enhances climate changes. Using walnut oil for hearty muffins is perfect for autumn, whereas using a light citrus olive oil can enhance a spring salad. And light olive oil paired with real butter is ideal for tea cookies, like this sweet and simple recipe that can be savored year-round just like tea.

While you decide which recipe and oils to try first, what better way than to make a batch of cookies, brew a cup of tea (black, green, white, or herbal), and make your decision(s). Thanks to olive oil proponent Gemma Sciabica, my baking buddy who has shown me the ropes of how to use liquid gold in cooking and baking. I like to use both olive oil and real butter (not margarine) for flavor when baking. The combination of oil and fat provides a crisp and moist cookie to write home about, especially when enjoying the soothing perks of tea.

1²⁄₃ cup flour
¾ teaspoon baking powder
⅛ teaspoon salt
⅓ cup butter or margarine, softened
⅓ cup granulated sugar
½ cup confectioners sugar
1½ teaspoons grated lemon peel

1½ teaspoons grated lime peel
3 tablespoons finely chopped fresh mint or 1 tablespoon finely chopped rosemary
¼ cup extra light olive oil
1 egg
Sugar (for dipping)

Mix flour, baking powder, and salt in a small mixing bowl; set aside. Cream butter, granulated sugar, confectioners sugar, lemon and lime peels, and mint in large mixing bowl. Blend in olive oil and egg. Stir in flour mixture. Cover and refrigerate for 1–2 hours. Preheat oven to 350°.

Shape dough into $3/5$-inch balls. Dip tops in sugar. Place balls 2 inches apart on ungreased baking sheet, sugared side up. Flatten to $1/8$-inch thickness with fork or bottom of drinking glass dipped in granulated sugar. Bake 7–11 minutes, or until cookies appear set in center. Carefully remove cookies from sheet immediately. Cool on wire rack.

(*Source:* North American Olive Oil Association)

THE GOLDEN SECRETS TO REMEMBER

✓ Mediterranean-type cooking includes nutrient-dense foods such as vegetables, fruits, grains, legumes, fish, poultry, and olive oil.

✓ There are countless olive oils to choose from when you are cooking, whether it is extra virgin olive oil, light olive oil, or flavored herb or citrus oils.

✓ Cooking sprays can help you be the best cook you can be.

✓ Storing your olive oils the right way will keep you and the people for whom you cook healthy and safe from oil that has expired.

✓ The Olive Oil Health-Boosting Five-Day Menu Plan is a sample of how you can incorporate heart-healthy and unforgettable olive oil–based recipes into your life— without going to Europe.

PART 7

OLIVE OIL RECIPES

Olive Oil Bon Appétit!

Looking back at the time on the Oregon coast as a dinner guest, when I didn't have a kitchen or a pot to boil in, to my years in graduate school, when I lacked culinary smarts—I've morphed. These days, I'm still a health nut, but now I can and do cook and bake in the comfort of my home for the health of it.

One late autumn, on an Indian summer type of afternoon, like an olive harvest, my kitchen pantry was full of olive oils from California to Umbria and an array of nut oils and tropical oils from around the world. I was home and ready to cook a feast for one. Fresh herbs and spices also were at hand, and after years I finally knew how to put them to work in harmony. A mixer (no more blender a quarter of a century old), pots, pans, and essential cookery surrounded me.

But that day, the time I was ready to whip up a meal, I was hit with life's challenges: One post-neutered pup that was ordered not to move for 14 days, one leak in the seam of my waterbed, one snowstorm, and one leaky filling to be filled. Instead of cooking an Herbed Roast Turkey (recipe in this book), I turned to healing oils and made one recipe at a time. To stave off stress eating and gaining 51 pounds in 2 days, I ate salads and vegetables drizzled with olive oil and rosemary flavored, fresh fruit chunks and nuts sweetened with coconut oil, and popcorn with grass-fed cow butter.

The Mediterranean diet is what I follow, but sometimes, like this time when Murphy's Law was a visitor, I followed a semi-Paleo diet—including vegetables and fruits and nuts. While I passed on whipping up the meal of the century, in retrospect it was olive oil and a variety of vegetable oils that helped keep me grounded and at peace, like a sturdy olive oil tree in a superstorm.

So, when life gains its normalcy (it does on its own time table), I'll hit the kitchen and whip up several dishes for guests that you'll find in this recipe section. And it was during this time of life's ups and downs that the epiphany welcomed me. Today, I could pass the Nutrition 101 class on oils and fats that I failed yesteryear—but it took me decades to do it.

Go ahead—visit this chapter often. You'll find a collection of tried and tested dishes that will take you to Olive Oil Land and other exotic places where other healing oils and fats are savored and enjoyed for their healing benefits and satisfaction of flavors.

Welcome to these original recipes for dozens of tasty delights, full of nutritious vegetables, fruits, fish, and poultry. These dishes, all tested, contain a variety of healthy oils. Many of these recipes also use garlic, onions and herbs.

For best results, use the olive oil brand mentioned in each recipe. However, feel free to use your own brand or another type of oil (such as canola oil). But note, Italian cook and olive oil guru Gemma Sciabica recommends using health-promoting extra virgin olive oil for *all* recipes.

Before you get started, I want you to first take the olive

oil quiz; discover epicurean enjoyment; and put to use must-have olive oil tips. Not only will you be eating a heart-healthy, anti-cancer Mediterranean-style diet, you'll be enjoying more taste and excitement in your meals as well as lifestyle for the rest of your life.

WHICH OLIVE OIL IS RIGHT FOR YOU?

Olive oil judges from coast to coast and around the world recognize award-winning olive oils, but despite their awards, some of these oils may not be a suitable match for you and your lifestyle. For instance, if you don't like mushrooms, porcini olive oil may not be your cup of oil. You may love to cook, but extra virgin olive oil may not give you enough pizzazz. Like to bake but don't want to be stuck using only canola oil (one healthful oil) for your breads, cakes, and muffins? You may be limiting yourself with your oil of choice.

No matter what kind of oil lover you are, take this quiz to get to know your personality and your real taste in oil before you choose the oil(s) for you.

Oils for Life

What's your lifestyle? Take this short quiz to find out.

1. A typical morning for you includes:
    A. Family chaos, with the dog joining in.
    B. Breakfast in bed.
    C. A 2-mile run.
    D. Computer work.
    E. Brunch at an ethnic restaurant.

2. When you cook, you like to:
    A. Feed a fun-loving crowd.
    B. Feed a loving mate or friend who enjoys your meals.
    C. Make a meal to take on the run.
    D. Make a low-maintenance meal.
    E. Work in a kitchen chock-full of exotic treats.

3. Your idea of a perfect vacation is:
    A. Grabbing the family and visiting relatives.
    B. Going to a secluded park for a picnic.
    C. Hitting the mountain trails.
    D. Enjoying an at-home movie fest with a few friends.
    E. Flying to a foreign country.

4. When the weekend hits, you can be found:
    A. Enjoying a family event with the in-laws, spouse, kids, cat, and dog.
    B. Busy with your hobbies.
    C. Jogging through the neighborhood.
    D. On the couch, cuddled up with you-know-who.
    E. Attending an out-of-town social event.

5. A meal to you means, in one word:
    A. Fun.
    B. Wholesome.
    C. Quick.
    D. Healthy.
    E. Exciting.

Tally Up

Once you understand your cooking and eating styles, you can use the knowledge to select oils that are compatible with them. This, in turn, will enhance your olive oil experience. See how you scored below. I've made a few oil-wise choices for you to get started or to add to your current olive oil repertoire.

Mostly A's: The Extrovert.

Your Style: You are well-rounded, fun-loving, and people-oriented. You want an oil that is versatile and good for kids and animals. An all-purpose olive oil is ideal. An oil that will not be too exotic during family get-togethers is best.

Your Best Oils: Extra virgin olive oil, roasted garlic olive oil, and citrus olive oils.

Mostly B's. The Introvert.

Your Style: You are the intellectual, an independent individual who may live alone. You'd probably enjoy an olive oil that is good for you and versatile, as opposed to strong-flavored.

Your Best Oils: Extra virgin olive oil, basil olive oil, and citrus olive oils.

Mostly C's. The Outdoor Health Nut.

Your Style: You are a physical person, ready to hike in the summer, hit the gym in the winter. You're an active individual with a sense of adventure as long as it's healthful.

Your Best Oils: Light olive oil, extra virgin olive oil, and porcini olive oil.

Mostly D's. The Indoor Hermit.

Your Style: You are a sofa spud, with one hand on the remote control and the other in a bag of wholesome doggie treats. An afternoon of baking is up your alley.

Your Best Oils: Extra virgin olive oil and homemade flavored olive oils.

Mostly E's. The Adventurer.

Your Style: You are ready to travel for work or play. Trying new foods is what life is all about. You enjoy tasting new foods and flavors wherever you go, and "bland" is not in your vocabulary.

Your Best Oils: Pepper olive oil, porcini olive oil, rosemary olive oil, and oregano olive oil.

EPICUREAN ENJOYMENT

The common trait of people who travel to Europe to enjoy the world of olive oil is that they know why this liquid gold is priceless. By listening to and learning from each and every olive oil buff, I have collected the following tips—about the traditional Mediterranean-type diet and lifestyle—which I now pass along to you to give you a taste of Tuscany:

1. Eat breakfast, and use olive oil in your frying pan and muffin tin.
2. Enjoy lunch, and don't hesitate to use a vinegar-and-oil dressing on fresh greens . . .
3. . . . And to dip your French bread into olive oil.
4. Say yes to fish at least two to three times per week.
5. Say no to processed foods. Think fresh, organic, and natural.
6. Incorporate physical activity into your everyday lifestyle—for your heart and your soul's sakes.
7. Pamper yourself, your family, and your pets with olive oil and olive oil–based beauty products, naturally.
8. Try olive oil as your first line of action to treat health ailments before using a traditional medicine.
9. Learn to fine-tune your taste buds to enjoy natural

foods, enhancing their flavors with Mother Nature's herbs and spices.

10. Chill and use olive oil and aromatic essential oils to de-stress and enjoy the wide world of olive oil mania.

Celeb chefs, olive oil–smart John Deane, M.D., and Dr. Seth Roberts, who turned to oil to maintain his weight, as well as the people at The Olive Press and the North American Olive Oil Association—and all the other unforgettable people in *The Healing Powers of Olive Oil*—get it. In their own individual ways, they understand that olive oil is an amazing folk medicine that is still embraced worldwide in the twenty-first century. You, like me and countless people around the world, can also reap the versatile benefits of olive oil without leaving home. Go ahead—enjoy the treasure that, after all these years, is still good as gold.

BEFORE YOU USE OLIVE OIL

You don't have to go to Spain, Italy, or Greece to enjoy the healing powers of olive oil. Whether you live on the West Coast, on the East Coast, in the Midwest, in the South, or in another country, you can find good local and imported olive oils that will bring you closer to achieving good health and well-being.

Keep in mind, however, that olive oil is not a magic bullet. Using it by itself or overindulging in the golden liquid to prevent or treat health ailments and lower your risk of disease isn't realistic.

Remember, the Mediterranean diet is more than just a diet. It is a lifestyle. By teaming meals based on vegetables, fruits, whole grains, fish, low-fat dairy products, and olive oil with daily physical activity, you can reap the healing benefits of the liquid gold and add years to your life.

When choosing an olive oil, remember to:

- Always check for the producing country's seal of authenticity—for instance, the COOC from California, the DOP from Italy, the AOC from France, the DOP from Greece, and the DO from Spain.
- Check the "use by" date.
- Check for winners of olive oil competitions. These olive oils will have seals, such as Gold, Silver, and Bronze medals, on their bottles.

FOUR SEASONS FOR SUPERFOODS WITH HEALING OILS

Winter

It's the Season: Every pre-winter in the Sierra, when the temperatures usually drop, I begin fantasizing about relocating to a place olive oil trees thrive. Perhaps it's the power outages, shoveling powder, and walking like a penguin on black ice that makes me crave healthful comfort food, including stir-fried dishes with tropical oils to southwestern fish salads and flavored citrus olive oils.

Winter Recipes: A cup of joe, warm ginger-lemon scones, and hearty poultry dishes provide winter with feel-good health perks. Comfort foods, including filling muffins, hit the spot when the days are shorter and nights are longer and colder.

Healing Oils: Olive oil, especially extra virgin olive oil, is used year-round. In the winter, it is often paired with all-purpose canola oil in baking and cooking. Herbal oils, including basil olive oil, oregano olive oil, and garlic olive oil are also used for hearty soups and stews. Hearty nut oils, such as walnut oil used for baking, is another healing oil that can appease the palate and make dishes flavorful.

Superfoods with Oil for Winter: Chocolate, cranberries, beans, carrots, fish, grapefruit, oats, oranges, tomatoes, and yogurt.

Ginger Lemon Oil Scones

❖ ❖ ❖

These scones are a perfect winter warming food. This recipe is for a whole, round, rustic ginger scone (not dropped ones or perfectly cut round ones). Scones can be healthy paired with honey and flavored olive oil. The chewy texture of candied ginger and a dusting of sugar is pretty in presentation and hearty for that colder season for mornings, snacks, or dessert.

2 cups all-purpose flour
1½ tablespoons baking powder
⅓ cup brown sugar
½ cup half-and-half or buttermilk
1 brown egg, beaten
2 tablespoons honey-flavored Greek yogurt
4 tablespoons European-style butter, (cold cubes)

*1 extra teaspoon, melted (for greasing pan)
2 tablespoons molasses
1 teaspoon ground ginger
2 tablespoons lemon-flavored olive oil
1 tablespoon fresh lemon rind
¾ cup crystalized ginger, finely chopped
Confectioners' sugar (for dusting)

In a mixing bowl, combine dry ingredients. Add butter-milk, egg, yogurt, and butter cubes. Stir in molasses, oil, ginger, and chopped ginger. Use a lightly greased round pan (I used a round, white tart dish). Bake at 375° for 30 minutes or until golden brown on top. Dust with sugar. This is a whole scone. Slice like a pie in half or quartered, and you'll have perfect triangle shapes. Makes 10–12. Serve warm with honey.

Eggplant Parmesan with Olive Oils

❖ ❖ ❖

Homestyle eggplant tastes better than the frozen stuff. You'll get less sodium and less fat than what you'll get at a restaurant. Pair servings with steamed artichokes (dip in half European-style butter and garlic-flavored olive oil) and enjoy eggplant heaven.

1 eggplant
1 tomato
Mediterranean sea salt
2 eggs, brown
1/8 cup 2 percent low-fat organic milk
1 cup bread crumbs (all
   natural with herbs)
1 tablespoon each extra virgin olive oil (fruity type)
   and basil olive oil

2 cups all-natural marinara
   sauce (with olive oil and
   garlic)
1 cup mozzarella cheese,
   skim, low-fat, grated
2 cups thin spaghetti whole
   grain pasta, cooked and
   drained
Parmesan cheese

Wash, drain, and slice eggplant into 1-inch circles. Sprinkle with salt; put in refrigerator for a few hours to prevent soggy slices. Combine egg and milk mixture. Dredge eggplant slices, and then dip both sides in bread crumbs. Place in a large frying pan with heated olive oils and brown on both sides. In a glass baking dish, layer eggplant slices, sauce, and mozzarella cheese. (The larger the dish, the better; this way the eggplant cooks evenly.) Bake at 350° for 30 to 40 minutes until bubbly and eggplant is tender. Meanwhile, in a saucepan, boil water and cook thin spaghetti al dente. Place eggplant slices on the side of pasta or on top. Garnish with fresh parmesan cheese. Serves 4.

Shepherd's Pie with Rosemary Olive Oil

❖ ❖ ❖

In my twenties, I was introduced to a taste of the mountain lifestyle, foreshadow of where I ended up decades later. After classes one chilly overcast day, a fellow student's friend invited me to his home. We drove on Highway 9 to his A-frame cabin in the Santa Cruz Mountains. I was charmed by the towering redwoods and the cozy fire he had made for ambiance while we enjoyed his dinner.

I asked, "What exactly is this dish called?" He answered, "Potato pie." He used russet potatoes, tomato sauce, and cheddar cheese. This peasant-style food was the only dish he knew how to make—but it was perfect. And that simple potato charmer (the down-to-earth potato dish, not the chef) became a friend for life during times of author famine and feast because I romanced it, and gave it a special flair with other ingredients.

4 yellow potatoes
¼ cup organic 2 percent
   low-fat milk
1 tablespoon European-style
   butter
Fresh chives
½ cup mushrooms, fresh,
   sliced
½ cup Roma tomatoes,
   chopped

¼ cup broccoli florets
2 tablespoons garlic olive oil
1 teaspoon Herbes De
   Provence
1¼ cup cheese mix, shred-
   ded (Monterey Jack,
   cheddar, asadero, queso
   quesadilla)
¼ teaspoon nutmeg
Fresh ground black pepper

In a large pot of water, place four washed potatoes. Boil until tender and rinse under cold water; peel skins. Put potatoes into a mixing bowl. Add milk, butter, and chives. Mash until smooth. Set aside. Sauté vegetables in olive oil. Add Herbes De Provence. Spread potatoes into a round 9 x 1½ inch pan or scalloped quiche dish. Top with vegetables. Sprinkle cheese on top. Bake at 350° for about 25 minutes or until cheese bubbles and top is slightly golden. Cool before slicing. Serves 6–8.

Trail Mix with Nut Oils

❖ ❖ ❖

Some people believe I live a boring life. And some people believe I eat a boring diet. But I know that nuts, seeds, and berries—part of the caveman diet—boast vitamins and minerals that are good for both the mind and body. Also, sometimes while indulging in the Mediterranean diet, I confess going overboard with dairy and bread. To stay lean and maintain my weight, I eat nuts, seeds, and berries—any form—to help me get back on track.

½ cup walnuts, chopped
½ cup cashews, lightly
   salted, halves
½ cup sunflower seeds,
   shelled
1 cup cranberries, dried

½ cup raisins
1 cup white chocolate chips
½ cup dark chocolate chips
2 tablespoons macadamia
   or walnut oil

In a large bowl, combine nuts, seeds, fruit, and chocolate. Mix well. Add nut oil. Pour mixture into a plastic container and cover with a lid. Store in refrigerator. Serves approximately 12.

This recipe takes less than a New York minute to put together. The bursts of winter colors like red, gold, brown, and white chips like snowdrops are handsome, especially when put into a glass container. I count on this energizing winter trail mix to be there during Old Man Winter to help me get through cold dog walks, swimming at the resort pool, dodging tourists, shoveling white powder, and bringing in the firewood to make a fire.

WARM UP TO WINTER BREAKFAST

The croissant, a French food, is a flaky roll cut in a crescent shape like a half-moon in pastry form. These little guys can be made from scratch, sold in bakeries, or in a tube ready to roll and bake—like I do in this recipe. Croissants can wrap sweet or savory fillings or cheese. This time around, I chose eggs and a buttery-style croissant. And putting this concoction together at home for breakfast is easy and warms the soul.

Continental Croissants

❖ ❖ ❖

4 organic brown eggs
4 slices Swiss cheese
½ cup organic 2 percent
* reduced fat milk*
1 tablespoon blend of
* canola and extra virgin*
* olive oil*
8 store-bought whole wheat
* crescent roll dough*

European-style butter
Parsley or basil and pepper
* to taste*
8 strips lean bacon
Honey
2 Roma tomatoes

In a bowl, beat eggs, cheese, and milk. Pour egg mixture into an oil-greased skillet. Over medium heat, make scrambled eggs (or an omelet). Set aside. Heat oven to 350°. Unroll dough and separate into triangles. Top each triangle with scrambled egg and cheese. Roll up as directed on can; shape into crescent pieces. Place on parchment paper–covered cookie sheet. Bake in a 350° oven for about 15 minutes or till golden brown. Spread tops with melted butter. Top with parsley or basil to taste. Keep warm. In another skillet, fry the bacon to crispy; drizzle with honey. Makes 8. Garnish with tomatoes. Serve with juice and coffee.

Winter Fruit Bowl: In a large bowl, mix 1 cup each of chopped apples, cranberries, oranges, and pears. Mix with a tablespoon of honey and lemon- or orange-flavored olive oil. Top with cinnamon and nutmeg. Chill. Serves 4–8.

Spring

It's the Season: When springtime rolls around, instead of racking up the extra winter sugar and calories, I make a switch and turn to lighter fare, including spring vegetables. During the seasonal change, it's time to spring clean and detox our bodies so we'll feel more energized, lose the muffin top, and feel healthier and happier.

Spring Recipes: When spring is in the air, baking doesn't have to be scratched. But dishes and their ingredients are lighter with seasonal fruits and vegetables. Healthy muffins, sandwiches, salads, and dessert foods are part of the lineup when snow turns to rain, and wildflowers and blossoming trees begin to welcome us to a renewed body and spirit.

Healing Oils: Spring is the time to bring out citrus oils, such as lemon-flavored and lime-flavored olive oils. Nut oils are lighter like peanut oil and sesame oil and are often used in vegetable stir-fry dishes—a welcome dish for lunch or dinner.

Superfoods with Oil for Spring: Crab, eggs, grapefruit, honey, kiwi, spinach, soy, strawberries, tea, and tofu.

Asian Honey Carrot Muffins

❖ ❖ ❖

These muffins are perfect for spring. I have a confession to make. I almost made a big bunny rabbit cake: A white cake with tart lemon filling, creamy buttercream frosting topped with coconut, jelly beans, and Peeps—yellow and pink. But I thought, "Why do I want to eat all that sugar?" So I chose hearty muffins with a carrot spin. I sense the Easter Bunny would be proud of me. This is my own recipe full of good-for-you ingredients.

2½ cups all-purpose whole
    wheat flour
2 teaspoons baking soda
2 teaspoons cinnamon
¼ teaspoon nutmeg
¼ teaspoon allspice
¼ teaspoon salt
½ cup honey
½ cup granulated sugar
½ cup brown sugar

3 brown eggs
½ cup extra light olive oil
1 tablespoon red palm oil
½ cup grass-fed butter
2½ cups shredded carrots
1 cup walnuts, chopped
½ cup raisins, amber
Raw honey (optional, for
    drizzling)

Heat oven to 350°. In a medium bowl, combine flour, baking soda, spices, and salt; set aside. In a small mixing bowl, combine the granulated and brown sugars, eggs, oils, and butter. Beat at high speed until creamy. Add the carrots and flour mixture. Mix on low speed to moisten. Blend on high speed for 1 minute, scraping the sides as needed. Stir in the walnuts and raisins. Pour into muffin tins. (I like the aluminum foil muffin holders. The size of muffins is your choice. The larger ones make more of an "oomph" impression, but if you're watching your weight, go smaller.) Bake 18–22 minutes or until the top springs back when touched lightly and a wooden pick inserted in the center comes out clean. Cool 10 minutes on the cooling racks. No frosting needed. Drizzle with raw honey if desired. Makes about 12 muffins.

Avocado Dip with Avocado Oil

❖ ❖ ❖

1 cup lemon Greek yogurt
½ cup sour cream
1 tablespoon honey (I used
    orange blossom)
2 tablespoons avocado oil

3 tablespoons fresh chives
2 tablespoons green onions,
    chopped
1½ cup baby carrots

In a bowl, combine yogurt, sour cream, honey, and oil. Fold in chives and onions. Put in fridge for an hour or two. Serve with organic carrots. Serves 4–6.

Garlic Oil Shellfish Combo

❖ ❖ ❖

Imagine: You're sitting in a popular restaurant at Fisherman's Wharf in San Francisco. On the second floor, your eyes feast on the panoramic view of the Golden Gate Bridge, boat marina, fishermen at work, and sea lions basking in the sun. A waiter serves you sourdough bread with pats of real butter and you sip ice water. You order a fresh Crab Louie combo. While waiting for your fresh fish meal, you're charmed by Mother Nature's ambiance at its finest. This is a picture-perfect scenario I experienced as a past resident of the San Francisco Bay Area.

Crab Louie is believed to have originated from San Francisco in the early 1900s. During nostalgic moments, I've enjoyed flashbacks of sea lions and crab salad. It was a sign for me to make my own Crab Louie combo. I learned that crab is not a budget-friendly fish. I also discovered crabs in shells aren't available on a whim. (I don't think it's in my animal-loving nature to boil live crabs or smash and shell dead ones. So there won't be a real-life amusing *Annie Hall* or *Julie and Julia* crustacean-type sequel for me to share.) It was meant to be to purchase the pricey, processed, and fresh-cooked Dungeness crab and precooked shrimp from the butcher at our friendly supermarket.

Keep in mind Dungeness crab is a tasty and healthful fish. The upside is it's protein rich, boasts heart-healthy vitamin B-12 and other essential nutrients, and it's low in saturated fat and calories. I was going to make the traditional Crab Louie dressing, but I went with oil and vinegar and topped the salad with it. I'm glad I did.

3 cups fresh spring mix
   salad (baby romaine,
   tango, radicchio)
2 brown eggs, hard-boiled
½ cup cherry tomatoes,
   sliced
½ cup cucumber, sliced
6–8 ounces Dungeness
   crab, cooked
3–4 ounces precooked baby
   shrimp, rinsed

4 tablespoons garlic olive
   oil (use extra for dipping
   French bread)
2 tablespoons red wine
   vinegar
Fresh lemon
Ground pepper to taste
Rosemary olive oil

In a large salad bowl, place a generous pile of greens. Top with eggs and vegetables (arrange in circle for a pretty and balanced presentation). Spoon the fish combo onto the middle of the salad. Serve oil and vinegar dressing in a small glass dish on the side. To add more flavors to your fish, use one tablespoon of fresh lemon juice and ground pepper. Serves 2.

To give this salad a twist, I serve warm sourdough bread drizzled with a bit of rosemary olive oil.

Hoagie with Extra EVOO

❖ ❖ ❖

This sandwich comes from Italian-American roots. As history tells it, the hero, or "hoagie," originated at Emil's Restaurant in South Philadelphia in the 1930s. It's been said that in Europe it would be a baguette, named after breads baked in European countries like Italy. Mediterranean salads often are made with fresh herbs, cheeses, and olive oil.

2 teaspoons of mayonnaise
   with olive oil
4 sourdough whole-wheat
   rolls or baguettes
4 slices provolone cheese
4 slices chicken or turkey
4 large Roma tomatoes,
   sliced
1 cup spinach lettuce,
   chopped

1 green bell pepper, sliced
¼ cup black olives, sliced
4 red onion slices
4 teaspoons extra virgin
   olive oil
Red wine vinegar to taste
Ground black pepper to
   taste

Spread mayo on warmed-up rolls, halved. Layer cheese and poultry. Top with vegetables. Drizzle with oil and vinegar. Sprinkle with pepper. Slice sandwiches diagonally. Serves 4.

Tropical Oil Bran Muffins

❖ ❖ ❖

A few years ago, I had a big affair with big muffins. After my swim at our hotel resort, I'd often buy a bag of Starbucks bran muffins and a cup of java. These days, I'm brewing my own coffee and making my muffins—smaller. This way, you get exactly what you want in size and ingredients—including healing oils—and the amazing taste and memorable aroma in your kitchen is worth the effort.

1 cup whole wheat flour
1 cup All Bran buds
1 tablespoon baking powder
3 tablespoons brown sugar
1 organic brown egg, beaten
½ cup reduced-fat butter-milk
¼ cup European-style butter

1½ cups fresh pineapple chunks
½ cup dark chocolate chips
1 tablespoon each, coconut and light olive oil
½ cup raisins
¼ cup coconut, shredded
2 tablespoons honey

In a bowl, combine dry ingredients. Add egg, buttermilk, butter, fruit, and chips. Use an ice-cream scoop to fill batter evenly into cupcake tins. Bake at 400° for about 25 minutes or until firm. Makes 12 medium-large muffins.

SUPER OILS FOR SPRING BRUNCH

I spent time spring cleaning, from vacuuming, dusting, washing windows, and tending to the ice patches on the deck—getting ready for a guest. I prepared appetizers, including a store-brought whole grain bread, a new bottle of olive oil, whole grain crackers, fresh vegetables, and herbal teas. I wanted to offer an ice-cream bunny cake, but I was the "health author," and she was into healing, so I passed. Then, when all was done, I waited and waited. Disappointed by her no-show, I felt sort of like I was waiting for the Easter Bunny that never came. I made a batch of Coconut Oil Ice-Cream Truffles. And after eating a couple, I felt like a kid and bounced back to going with the flow. The upside: I enjoyed a clean home and was stocked with clean food.

Coconut Oil Ice-Cream Truffles

❖ ❖ ❖

14 ounces all-natural chocolate ice cream

14 ounces all-natural coffee ice cream

2 tablespoons 2 percent organic reduced-fat milk

2 tablespoons virgin coconut oil

1 cup white chocolate chips

1 cup sweetened flaked coconut

½ cup pecans, chopped

Set aside a rectangular pan lined with parchment paper. Take ¼ to ½ cup of ice cream, make six balls each of vanilla and coffee ice cream, and place in pan. Cover with foil and freeze for several hours to form a round shape. When ready to make truffles, melt chocolate in the microwave. Let sit until cool; roll each ball into milk, oil, and chocolate (use your hands). Then roll in coconut and nuts. Place each truffle back on the pan. Freeze till firm and serve on pastel-colored plates. Serves 6.

Yogurt and ice cream provide calcium and protein, and both avocado oil and coconut oil are plentiful in monounsaturated fats. That means, you'll feel satisfied and not be tempted to overindulge. Sometimes things happen the way we plan. But these recipes are fail-proof and will be there for you if visitors knock on the door or are a no-show. Another cool thing about these two easy-to-make springtime treats is that they're fun to make and won't pack on unwanted pounds for the upcoming season.

Summer

It's the Season: When summertime rolls around, no-cook meals, cold foods, and picnics come with the territory. I do like the summer, too, especially in the Sierra with its warm temperatures and unpredictable lightning and thunderstorms—and light healthful cooking with healthy cooking oils.

Summer Recipes: Hotter weather and more time to be out-doors leads to cold cereals, grilled fish, poultry, pasta dishes, sandwiches, smoothies, and salads.

Healing Oils of the Summer: Olive oil and light olive oil are mainstays during summer as are herbal olive oils including garlic-flavored olive oil, and jalapeño-flavored olive oil. These flavorful oils add a punch to cold salads, dips, and sauces.

Superfoods of the Summer: Avocado, blackberries, blueberries, celery, garlic, lettuce, peaches, salmon, strawberries, and yogurt.

Rustic Strawberry Galette

❖ ❖ ❖

Meet a galette. It is a flat, round, open-face type of pastry or pie popular in French cuisine. It can be filled with summer fruit—berries—and made sweeter with a glaze. A rustic fruit galette has a mountain feel to it—and I fell into making it during the warmer days of summer. The pie crust called out to me "I'm free form." And I decided to go with the flow and made my first one.

1 store-bought premium pie crust

2–3 cups strawberries, firm, sliced

¼ cup granulated sugar (you can use less)

2 teaspoons cinnamon

2 tablespoons European-style butter

1 tablespoon of half-and-half

¼ cup organic apricot or strawberries preserves

1 tablespoon lemon-flavored olive oil

Preheat oven to 350°. Take out refrigerated pie dough; unroll the circle on a parchment-paper-lined cookie sheet.

Fold dough edges over so it looks like a swimming pool or hot tub liner. Fill with berry slices. Sprinkle with sugar, cinnamon, and dabs of butter. Brush edges with half-and-half. Bake about 50 minutes till filling is bubbly and crust is golden brown.

About 10 minutes after the galette has cooled, nuke apricot preserves and lemon-flavored olive oil in microwave till warm; spread on top of strawberries. Cool. Put in refrigerator for a few hours to firm. Cut like a pie. Serves 8.

Chunky Tomato Guacamole with Chips

❖ ❖ ❖

This recipe is my own, one that evolved from my first attempts at guacamole creations in the Santa Cruz Mountains during the summertime. During this chapter of my life, I was a grad student living on a shoestring budget and only had enough money to buy avocadoes and store-bought salsa in a bottle. These days, I can tell you that making your own guacamole with fresh ingredients is not pricey and worth the effort.

2 ripe avocadoes
½ green chili pepper, chopped
3 tablespoons fresh onion (yellow or red), chopped
2 tablespoons garlic, chopped
1 tablespoon fresh lemon juice
2 Roma tomatoes
Ground pepper to taste
Parmesan cheese, fresh and grated

Slice two avocados in half. Scoop into a medium-sized bowl; mash with a fork. Add chili pepper, onion, and garlic. Mix lightly. Add juice and tomatoes. Season to taste, top with cheese, and cover bowl with a top. Put in refrigerator to chill.

BAKED TORTILLA CHIPS WITH OLIVE OIL

4 to 6 100 percent whole
    wheat tortillas, soft taco
    size
2 tablespoons extra virgin
    olive oil, lemon flavored

Ground pepper and
    Mediterranean
    sea salt to taste

Preheat oven to 350°. Slice tortillas in half three times (like slicing a pie) so you have six triangle-shaped pieces for each. Place in rectangular baking pan. Brush with olive oil. Bake for about 10 minutes. Remove from oven and place in ceramic bowl. Sprinkle with spice. Serve warm with cold chunky tomato guacamole dip. Makes 3–4 servings.

Coconut Oil Granola Supreme

❖ ❖ ❖

¾ cup sweetened coconut
2 cups rolled oats (instant or
    old fashioned, the latter
    preferred)
1 teaspoon ground cinna-
    mon
¼ teaspoon freshly ground
    ginger
½ cup honey (orange
    blossom)

¼ cup grass-fed butter,
    unsalted
½ cup almonds, sliced
2 tablespoons coconut oil
2 tablespoons extra virgin
    olive oil
1 teaspoon pure vanilla ex-
    tract
1 cup golden raisins

On a parchment-lined cookie sheet, spread coconut. Bake at 375° till lightly toasted. Set aside. Turn down oven to 350°. In a bowl, combine oats and spices. Pour mixed honey, butter, oils, and vanilla. Place mixture on parchment-lined cookie sheet or pan. Bake approximately 30 minutes. Mix occasionally. Cool. Mix in coconut and almonds. Store in container and keep in refrigerator. Add dried fruit such as pineapple or crystallized ginger. Eat as a cereal or energy snack.

Tacos with an Olive Oil Twist

❖ ❖ ❖

There is something special and comforting about creating a meatless dish with natural cheese and vegetables. The taste of onions and butter with flavored olive oil will wow your taste buds and help you chase away unwanted weight because it will fill you up not out.

12 Roma tomatoes, chopped	*4 chilies, minced*
½ cup red onion, chopped	*A dash of Mediterranean sea salt and pepper*
4 whole wheat flour tortillas	*2 teaspoons extra virgin olive oil*
1 teaspoon lime-flavored olive oil	*1 cup cheese (a blend of four Mexican types)*
1 teaspoon European style butter	*Extra lime-flavored olive oil for drizzling*
1 cup organic baby spinach	

In a bowl, place tomatoes, chilies, onion, olive oils, and spices. Put in refrigerator for about an hour to chill for a better flavor. In a skillet, heat a bit of butter. Place one tortilla in it for about one minute until it bubbles and turn over. Repeat. Sprinkle cheese on it and fold over till cheese is melted. Remove. Repeat. Top with lettuce and salsa. Drizzle with lime-flavored olive oil for a citrusy twist. Makes 4 tacos.

Peachy Muffins with Canola Oil

❖ ❖ ❖

1¾ cups all-natural 100 percent whole wheat flour
1 cup quick cooking oats
½ cup dark brown sugar
2 tablespoons baking powder
¼ teaspoon baking soda
1 large brown egg, beaten
¼ cup European-style butter, softened
2 tablespoons canola oil

2 tablespoon extra virgin olive oil
1½ cups fresh peaches, chopped
1 cup 2 percent low-fat organic milk
½ cup walnuts or pecans, chopped
1 teaspoon pure vanilla extract
Organic raw sugar to taste
1 teaspoon allspice

In a bowl, combine dry ingredients (whole wheat flour, oats, baking powder, baking soda, brown sugar); in another bowl, mix milk and oats, soak for 15 minutes. (This is a great tip that makes the oatmeal not gritty.) Add beaten egg, soft butter, and oils. Fold in peaches (I leave the skins on), vanilla, and allspice. Use a ½ cup ice-cream scoop for big muffins and pour into lined cupcake tins. Sprinkle each muffin with sugar for a nice crunch. Bake at 400° for 15–20 minutes until golden brown. Makes 12 muffins.

Fries by the Sea

I've had a love affair with French fried potatoes since I was a kid. You don't need to be a child or French chef to know that fries are served hot and savored as a snack or served with other food for lunch or dinner. Every time I enjoy an order of this finger food it takes me back to a favorite seaside town.

Enter Monterey. Years ago, to prepare for my SFSU oral exams on authors, I paid a visit to the Salinas Library to study works of one of my favorites: John Steinbeck. (He stayed at Fallen Leaf Lake one winter, snowbound with two dogs.) I was tucked away solo in a room for more than 12 hours as I went through the master's works including a backdrop of Monterey. After my research, on an overcast day, I recall strolling through Cannery Row, a place Steinbeck wrote about. I ordered fries, served in one of those red plastic baskets, and dipped each French fry into ketchup while feeling the ocean air feed the senses: sight, smell, and scent. I've missed the coastal town, bit I discovered how I can bring it to me.

Olive Oil and Sea Salt Fries

❖ ❖ ❖

2 extra-large Russet potatoes with skins, cut lengthwise
Ground pepper and sea salt to taste
1-2 teaspoons European-style butter

Natural malt vinegar
1 tablespoon garlic olive oil
2 teaspoons fresh parsley (garnish)

Preheat oven to 450°. Place potato wedges on a parchment-lined cookie sheet. Pour butter and oil over potatoes. Sprinkle with salt and pepper. Bake about 25 minutes or until golden brown and crispy. Turn at least once. Drizzle with malt vinegar and garnish parsley on top. Put fries on a plate or wicker basket lined with a white napkin. Best when served fresh and hot right out of the oven. Serves 2.

I've devoured countless bags of vinegar and sea salt potato chips, but never served fries with vinegar. On Tuesday afternoon for a snack when it was cold and rainy, I made a batch of home fries. This recipe calls for premium ingredients, including the best Russet potatoes, malt vinegar (pricey but worth it), and sea salt, not the regular stuff. These fries are easy to make and bake. The big homemade taste is worth the small effort. Olive Oil and Sea Salt Fries are good food by the sea—a place dear to the unforgotten author and me, another lover of writing, water, and canines.

Fall

It's the Season: When I migrated to Tahoe, the first autumn in 1999, it was a big change from the San Francisco Bay Area. I was welcomed with leaves changing color— hues of red, orange, and yellow—and aspen trees vibrant gold. The pinecones from the towering pine trees dropped onto the ground with pine needles (from gusty winds and a thunderstorm or two). Busy squirrels were hither and thither, plus colder nights (temperatures in the twenties) minus vegetable and fruit stands along the sides of major highways.

Fall Recipes: In the Sierra, Pacific Northwest, Deep South, and Northeast to the Midwest, autumn is a time of year when pumpkin and sweet potatoes come into play, as well as cooking hearty soups and casseroles—all can be enhanced with cooking oils.

Healing Fall Oils: Late September until late December is the season for warming foods paired with olive oil to an array of healing oils that give pizzazz to baking, casseroles, sautéing, and stews. Oils that come into play during autumn include all olive oils for cooking; light olive oil, canola oil, and coconut oil for baking; herbal-flavored oil for dipping/drizzling, stir-fries; citrus-flavored oils for poultry; and nut oils for baking cakes to cookies.

Superfoods of the Fall: Apples, broccoli, cauliflower, cranberries, oats, oranges, pumpkin, sweet potatoes, turkey, and walnuts.

Cranberry Orange Walnut Oil Muffins

❖ ❖ ❖

One Thanksgiving, someone asked me if turkey dinner was part of my week.

My answer was, "I'm not sure."

If by "turkey dinner" you mean cooking a big bird and making dressing, potatoes, greens, and pecan pie, then the answer is no.

Which reminds me of a past nontraditional November holiday story.

I was a journalist living in the San Francisco Bay Area, on deadline writing three articles for a national women's magazine. Unfortunately, it was raining cats and dogs and I caught a miserable cold. Like a trooper, I took my former Brittany down the stairs of my rustic bungalow, outside into the pouring rain and into my garage-converted study. Working late into the night by candlelight amid intermittent power outages, I was interrupted by a light knock on the wooden door. It was Virginia, my landlady, an octogenarian woman who was my surrogate grandmother with European roots and a heart of gold.

A short, plump woman with facial wrinkles of experience, she handed me a large bag. Inside it was a care package complete with roasted turkey from the deli, oranges, dried cranberries, walnuts, packaged greens with a bottle of vinegar and olive oil, sore throat lozenges, and bottled water. I was moved, and grateful for her generosity. And thanks to the Good Samaritan, I finished each article and pleased my editor; I survived the cold. One week later, my dear friend was home sick with a cold. She called me requesting a few wellness items from the store. Without hesitation, I whipped up Cranberry Orange Walnut Oil Muffins and while they were baking, got the goods, including orange juice, cough syrup, and aspirin. When I delivered the bag of goods to my "Gran," she gave me a slight smile. No words needed. I got it. It was the gift of gratitude.

2¼ cups all-purpose flour
 (¼ is for high altitude) (if
 preferred, use half whole
 wheat flour)
1½ teaspoons baking powder
1 teaspoon baking soda
1 tablespoon honey
¼ cup brown sugar
⅔ cup fresh premium
 orange juice (pulp, not
 concentrated)
¾ cup low-fat buttermilk
1 organic brown egg

2 tablespoons European-
 style butter, softened
1 tablespoon walnut oil
1 tablespoon orange-
 flavored olive oil
1 cup dried cranberries
½ cup walnuts, chopped
1 teaspoon orange zest
Olive oil to grease loaf pan
Fresh cranberries for
 garnish
Clover honey

In a large bowl, combine dry ingredients (flour, baking powder, baking soda). Stir in honey, juice, buttermilk, egg, butter, and walnut and olive oils. Fold in berries, nuts, and zest. Lightly grease (with olive oil or butter) muffin tins (or a 9-x-5-inch loaf pan). Bake at 350° for about 50–60 minutes or until firm and golden brown. Cool. Serve with clover honey (lemon cream honey adds a nice kick) or butter. Serves approximately 12.

This fruit-nut bread is a gift of good health. Both fruit and nuts go back to the beginning of time. The contrast of sweet and tart flavors from the fresh cranberries and citrus, and meaty crunch of nuts is good and the moist texture is better. A Cranberry Orange Walnut Oil muffin spread with honey and paired with a cup of hot black or green tea or gourmet coffee (cinnamon spice or French vanilla is nice for autumn) will boost your mental and physical powers. Simply use the burst of energy to recall who you're thankful for and pay it forward.

Macadamia Nut Oil Cookies

❖ ❖ ❖

1 cup European-style butter
2 capfuls macadamia nut oil
½ cup confectioners sugar, premium brand
½ cup macadamia nuts, ground fine (I used a coffee grinder)
2 capfuls pure vanilla extract
2¼–2½ cups unbleached all-purpose flour (for tradition's sake)

Approximately ¾ cup confectioners sugar (for rolling)
Optional: Dark chocolate chips, finely chopped (for inside cookies)
Optional: Orange and chocolate sprinkles for fall and/or Halloween

In a mixing bowl, cream butter, oil, and sugar until smooth and blended well. Add nuts (almost like a paste) and vanilla. Cup by cup, add flour, and mix until it's dough. Chill for 30 minutes. Use a plastic tablespoon to form dough into a uniform round ball, (use your hands) and place dough balls on an ungreased cookie sheet. (Tip: Try a test cookie to ensure you used enough flour. It could vary depending on your environment and you may need to use a bit more. Cookies should not spread but stay true to ball shape.)

Bake at 350° for 12–15 minutes. Do not overbake. Roll in confectioners sugar when warm and again when cool. Makes 22–24 cookies. (Caveat: These petite cookies are decadent and addictive! You don't want to overindulge in sugar or butter, so share or freeze for a snow day or holiday.)

Sweet Potato Pie with Lemon Oil

❖ ❖ ❖

3 cooked organic sweet potatoes, mashed well

2 organic brown eggs

½–1 cup brown sugar

¾ cup organic half-and-half

¼ cup unsalted (or European-style) butter, melted

2 teaspoons lemon olive oil

1 tablespoon all-purpose flour (or whole wheat)

2 teaspoons pure vanilla extract

2 teaspoons ground cinnamon

1 teaspoon pumpkin spice

Pinch of sea salt

1 tablespoon nutmeg

1 store-bought premium pie shell (or olive oil crust, see Chapter 9, "Combining Olive Oil and Vinegar")

Honey, (for garnish) whipped cream

Walnuts, chopped (for garnish)

In a mixing bowl, combine potatoes, eggs, sugar, half-and-half, butter, vanilla, and oil. Beat until smooth. Add flour, cinnamon, sea salt, and pumpkin spice. Pour mixture into homemade or precooked pie shell (follow directions and wrap foil around the edges so they don't overcook). Sprinkle with nutmeg. Bake at 375° for about 1 hour or until toothpick comes out clean, which indicates pie is firm. Cool. Drizzle with honey, top with a dollop of whipped cream and walnuts. Serves 8–10.

While savoring a piece of warm pie fresh out of the oven, enjoy the rich flavors from its sweet food companions. As a Northern California native, I admit I miss the companionship of pals with artsy dreams. It was my goal to become a writer. While I would love to get a blast from the past (and share a pie with my all-grown-up down-to-earth friends), I wouldn't give up my kitchen complete with a stainless-steel mixer, baking utensils, and serene study amid a mountain setting in the fall. It's sweet.

Olive Oil Pumpkin Squares

❖ ❖ ❖

On Turkey Day the traditional meal includes a big bird, dressing, potatoes, greens—and pumpkin pie, my favorite part of the meal. This year, I spiced up the popular round pie recipe and gave it a different shape, more spice, and a twenty-first-century sweet spin for the thrill of taste and presentation. Several years ago, I whipped up a nontraditional dinner for Thanksgiving. On the menu was pasta with marinara sauce and turkey meatballs, garlic French bread, and a Greek green salad with feta cheese and tomatoes drizzled with olive oil and red wine vinegar. I did give in to tradition and served a store-bought pumpkin pie, the kind found in the frozen food aisle.

I served this meal of Mediterranean-type dishes to my sibling. I was happy (the family pictures show me smiling), but he was a bit turned off (as were my bird dogs; their pics are nondescript) because there was no bird, no leftovers. Worse, the pie was a bit boring. After dinner I played the classic Hitchcock film *The Birds* for comic relief, but I was on my own before the lovebird pet-shop scene. Years later, I tried my hand at creating a new, improved pumpkin pie dessert. I'm not sure what I'll be cooking for the event, but these squares upstage the "normal" pie.

Spicy pumpkin pie squares upstage a triangle slice of pie big time. Not only does the cute shape turn heads, but the sweet topping provides a creamy and crunchy bit that's yummy. The double crust on the bottom gives the squares a thick, cobbler-like, chewy crust texture. After trying this recipe, you may never go back to the round pumpkin pie. The redo is easy and boasts rustic charm with the double crust, cream, and cookie crunch.

1 15-ounce can pumpkin puree
2 organic brown eggs
½–¾ cup brown sugar
1 cup organic half-and-half
½ cup organic 2 percent low-fat milk
1 tablespoon honey
1 teaspoon fresh ginger, minced

2 teaspoons pure vanilla extract
2 teaspoons pumpkin spice
1 teaspoon nutmeg
1 tablespoon extra virgin olive oil or butter
2 store-bought roll-out pie crusts

HONEY TOPPING

*Whipped cream, Greek
    yogurt, or honey to taste*
½ cup store-bought ginger

*cookies, chopped into
    crumbs*

In a mixing bowl, combine pumpkin puree, eggs, sugar, half-and-half, milk, and honey. Beat until smooth. Add vanilla, ginger, and pumpkin spice. Pour mixture into 8-x-8-inch oil or butter greased square baking dish lined with two layered pie crusts. Flute edges around the square dish (it shouldn't be perfect for a home-style effect). Sprinkle top with nutmeg. Cover pie crust edges with foil to cook evenly. Bake at 375° for about 50 minutes or until knife comes out clean, which indicates pie is firm. Cool. Cut into squares. Drizzle with honey; top with a dollop of whipped cream and ginger cookie (crisp but not hard) crumbs. Serves 9–12.

Taco Salad with Avocado Oil

❖ ❖ ❖

*¼ cup tomatoes, sliced and
    chopped*
*2 cups mixed greens, pre-
    washed, dark, preferred*
*½ cup provolone cheese,
    grated or cut in thin
    slices*
¼ cup avocado, sliced
¼ cup black olives, sliced

*¼ cup sunflower seeds,
    shelled*
2 teaspoons avocado oil
*½ cup salsa (see recipe
    below)*
¼ cup sour cream
*Tortilla chips (see recipe
    below)*

In a large salad bowl, mix tomatoes with greens. Fold in cheese, avocado, olives, and seeds. Drizzle with avocado oil.

Top with salsa and sour cream. Surround with tortilla chips. Serves 2.

CHUNKY HOT SALSA

2 Roma tomatoes, chopped
¼ cup red onion, diced

½ chili green pepper, diced
½ teaspoon lemon olive oil

In a small bowl, mix tomatoes, onion, and pepper. Drizzle olive oil on top. Mix and chill. Serves 1–2.

BAKED TORTILLA CHIPS

2 whole grain tortillas, sliced in triangle shapes

1 teaspoon European-style butter
1 teaspoon olive oil

Place triangle-shaped tortilla pieces in a pan. Place butter and oil on top. Bake at 375° for about 10–15 minutes until light golden brown. Serve warm. Serves 1–2.

Cookies with Nut Oil

❖ ❖ ❖

Back in 2007, I was a frequent player of Wheel of Fortune slot machines. I had a winning formula. Once I got that win-win feeling, I'd grab my swimsuit and hit the casinos. Then, walking around the dollar slots, if I got a good vibe I knew it was the right machine. One weekday in five minutes I won four hundred bucks and cashed out. In the snow, I swam, hit the hot tub, and treated myself to a Starbucks big peanut butter cookie. It was heaven.

As a kid, my mom's peanut butter cookies turned out—

mine did not. I didn't follow directions. After trial and error, throughout the years, I combined peanut butter with chocolate. What's more, I used both butter and nut oils, and spices to give these cookies a Mediterranean flair.

Double Peanut Butter Cookies

❖ ❖ ❖

2½ cups all-natural whole wheat flour
¾ cup light brown sugar
2 organic brown eggs
1 teaspoon almond oil
1 teaspoon peanut oil
¾ cup creamy peanut butter (not old-fashioned)
⅜ cup European-style butter

2 teaspoons pure vanilla extract
1 teaspoon allspice
Pinch of Mediterranean sea salt
1 cup white chocolate chips
1 cup dark chocolate chips
½ cup peanuts, chopped

In a bowl, combine flour, sugar, eggs, almond oil, peanut oil, peanut butter, and butter. Add vanilla, spice, and salt. Fold in chocolate chips, and peanuts. Chill for 1 hour. Roll dough into 1-inch balls (I put a bit of peanut butter in the middle of each for an extra punch) and place on parchment-lined cookie sheet. With a fork, make crisscross imprints if preferred. Bake at 375° for about 10 minutes or until golden brown. Makes 30 medium-sized cookies.

The cookies fresh out of the oven smelled of peanut butter and the aroma in my kitchen felt warm and inviting. Mixing chocolate is a delight because you get the best of both worlds if you're a chocolate lover. Teaming a few homemade cookies with a cup of hot antioxidant-rich green tea is like hitting the feel-good jackpot.

Breakfast

In my twenties, I didn't believe in breakfast. But today, I can still hear my mom nag, "You should eat a bowl of cereal and a piece of fruit. It will give you energy for the day and keep you healthier as you grow up." It turns out Mom was right. So are all those breakfast-loving Europeans in the Mediterranean countries. Italians, Greeks, and Spaniards take time out for breakfast.

And these days, I do savor this meal, whether I'm at work or play at home, on a book tour, or out in the field doing research for a book. The fact is, breakfast is the most important meal of the day because it can rev up your metabolism and keep you burning calories all day long. This is key to staying lean and maintaining your ideal weight.

So, I have gotten into the habit of eating oatmeal, fruit, fresh orange juice, low-fat or nonfat yogurt, and coffee with low-fat milk. On special days (such as in a hotel room or on a Sunday morning at home), I do love special treats such as healthful muffins or pancakes. But, rather than turn to tasty treats that have a long list of ingredients that you can't pronounce, make your own scrumptious breakfast goodies. Here, take a look at some tasty, good-for-you recipes worth writing home to Mom about.

Blueberry Pancakes
Apple Nut Oil Muffins
Italian EVOO Omelet
Pumpkin Lemon Oil Waffles

Blueberry Pancakes

❖ ❖ ❖

1½ cups flour
¼ cup sugar
1 tablespoon baking powder
½ teaspoon baking soda
½ teaspoon salt
1¾ cups buttermilk

⅓ cup ricotta cheese
2 tablespoons Marsala
   Olive Oil
2 eggs
2 cups blueberries

In a mixing bowl, combine the dry ingredients. Make a well in the center and pour in buttermilk, ricotta, olive oil, and eggs. Stir just until the mixture is moistened. Fold in the blueberries. Lightly oil a griddle or large non-stick skillet over medium heat. Drop the batter by ¼ cups onto the hot griddle and spread gently into 4-inch rounds. Cook the pancakes 2–3 minutes. Turn the pancakes over and cook 1–2 more minutes. Repeat with the remaining batter. Place the pancakes on a cookie sheet and keep them warm in the oven while cooking the remaining batter. Serve them with blueberry sauce or pure maple syrup.

(*Source: Baking Sensational Sweets with California Olive Oil* by Gemma Sanita Sciabica)

Apple Nut Oil Muffins

❖ ❖ ❖

These muffins take me back to my starving student days in San Jose as an undergrad. One special day in my favorite creative writing class, I asked my professor, "Do I have any talent? I want to be a writer." My heart raced as I waited eagerly for her response as if she were a psychic. She answered, "You should move on to San Francisco State University. That is where you need to be." I gave her a muffin; she gave me incentive to move on, as the author did for the 16-year-old aspiring writer in the film *Finding Forrester*. This is a sweet, revamped recipe of mine—a gift from me to you.

$\frac{1}{2}$ cup packed light brown sugar

2 teaspoons baking powder

$\frac{1}{4}$ teaspoon baking soda

$\frac{1}{2}$ teaspoon sea salt (optional)

$1\frac{1}{2}$ cups whole wheat flour

1 brown egg, lightly beaten

$\frac{1}{4}$ cup light olive oil

1 teaspoon walnut oil

1 teaspoon cinnamon oil

1 teaspoon European-style butter

$\frac{1}{2}$ cup sour cream

2 capfuls pure vanilla extract

$\frac{1}{4}$ cup orange juice, not concentrated, with pulp

$1\frac{1}{2}$ cups apples (Fuji or Granny Smith), peeled and cut into small cubes

$\frac{1}{2}$ cup walnuts, chopped

Raw sugar for topping

Line 12 muffin tins with paper liners. In a bowl, combine sugar, baking powder, baking soda, and salt. Add flour. In another bowl, combine egg, olive oil, walnut oil, cinnamon oil, butter, sour cream, vanilla, and orange juice. Mix all ingredients. Fold in apples and nuts. Spoon batter with an ice-cream scoop into muffin tins (I used yellow and green liners for fall). Sprinkle with sugar and bake approximately 18–20 minutes at 350°. Makes 12 muffins.

Italian EVOO Omelet

❖ ❖ ❖

Eggs in moderation are part of the heart-healthy Mediterranean diet. The scent of garlic and onion teamed with hot, cheesy eggs with tomatoes and mushrooms is hearty, comforting, and filling with its mixture of flavors—and it's easy to make. Plus, omelets are budget friendly.

2 tablespoons extra virgin
   olive oil
3 large brown eggs, beaten
1 tablespoon red onion,
   chopped
2 tablespoons half-and-half
½ teaspoon garlic, minced

½ cup Romano tomato,
   chopped
¼ cup mushrooms, sliced
½ cup cheddar cheese,
   grated
Black pepper to taste
Parsley (for garnish)

In a medium-sized frying pan, sauté garlic, onion, tomato, and mushrooms in 1 tablespoon of oil. In a bowl, beat eggs, add half-and-half. Over medium heat, pour egg and milk mixture into another hot nonstick 8-inch round skillet with 1 tablespoon of olive oil. Cook for a few minutes until egg firms. Use spatula to lift edges of omelet. Top half of the omelet with vegetables, onion, garlic, and cheese. Fold in half, then put lid on pan for a few minutes until egg is light brown and cheese is melted. Place omelet on plate. Garnish with sprinkled cheese, parsley, and pepper. Makes 1 or 2 servings.

Pumpkin Lemon Oil Waffles

❖　❖　❖

1 cup whole wheat flour
1½ teaspoons baking powder
¾ teaspoon nutmeg
1 teaspoon ground cinnamon

2 organic brown eggs
3 tablespoons honey
½ cup pumpkin puree
1 tablespoon olive oil
1 tablespoon lemon-flavored olive oil

TOPPING

2 tablespoons honey
Confectioners sugar for dusting (optional)

2 tablespoons butter
1 cup fresh berries

In a mixing bowl, combine flour, baking powder, nutmeg, and cinnamon. In a smaller bowl, stir eggs and honey. Pour into dry ingredients. Add pumpkin. Mix well. Turn on non-stick waffle iron. Pour half of batter onto hot iron; close. Wait until steam rises. Remove waffles and top with sugar, butter, honey, and berries. Makes 2 servings. (Double the recipe for friends and family.)

Appetizers and Breads

An appetizer doesn't have to be fattening or unhealthy. Plenty of appetizers, such as these Mediterranean types, can include fresh vegetables, garlic, nuts, and olive oil. At Frantoio's Restaurant in Mill Valley, California, the menu includes an array of irresistible appetizers that each are fit for a meal by itself.

Not only will appetizers such as slices of warm homemade Olive Bread dipped in fresh extra virgin olive oil give you an Italian taste, they will curb your hunger pangs so you won't be tempted to overeat at lunch or dinner. And note, while dinner can be nutritious and delightful, to people who follow a true Mediterranean diet, it is the lightest meal of the day and eaten before 7:00 P.M. Appetizers like these can help you stay on track.

-----

100 Percent Whole Wheat Loaf
Orange Olive Bread
Stuffed Eggs

-----

100 Percent Whole Wheat Loaf

❖ ❖ ❖

Most whole wheat bread you buy at the supermarket is, in fact, white bread with just a smidgen of whole wheat flour and a lot of added color and chemicals. Then, many folks try to bake their own whole wheat bread at home—often with limited success. If your experience with homemade 100 percent whole wheat bread is a loaf that's heavy and dry, with a slightly bitter undertone, this recipe will change your mind.

1½ cups (12 ounces)
  water
¼ cup sunflower seeds,
  chopped
3 tablespoons (1¼ ounces)
  olive oil
5 tablespoons (3¾ ounces)
  honey, molasses, or
  maple syrup

¼ cup (⅛ ounce) walnuts,
  chopped
1½ teaspoons salt
3½ cups (14 ounces) whole
  wheat flour
1½ teaspoons instant yeast
1 tablespoon whole grain
  bread improver
  (optional)

In a large mixing bowl, or in the bowl of an electric mixer, combine all the ingredients, mixing to form a shaggy dough. Let the dough rest for 20 minutes, which gives the flour a chance to absorb the liquids, then knead it for about 10 minutes, until it's smooth and supple. The dough will seem very wet and slack at first; just keep mixing and eventually it will come together, though it will remain sticky. Note: For optimal rise, use either a bread machine (set on the dough setting) or an electric mixer to mix and knead this dough, with the bread machine being the first choice; kneading by hand will result in a smaller, denser loaf.

Let the dough rise, in a greased, covered bowl, for 1 hour. Shape it into a log and place it in a lightly greased 8½-x-4½-inch bread pan. Cover the pan (with a proof cover or lightly greased plastic wrap) and let it rise for about 1 hour, until it has crowned about 2 inches over the rim of the pan.

Preheat the oven to 350°. Bake the bread for 45 minutes, tenting it lightly with aluminum foil for the final 20 minutes of baking. Remove from the oven, turn it out of the pan, and cool it on the rack.

(*Source: The King Arthur Flour Baker's Companion: The All-Purpose Baking Cookbook*)

Orange Olive Bread

❖ ❖ ❖

¼ cup Sciabica's or
  Marsala extra virgin
  olive oil
3 cups flour
1 cup orange juice
1 tablespoon sugar or honey

1 package dry yeast
1 teaspoon salt (or to taste)
6 black olives, chopped
1 tablespoon fresh
  rosemary, finely chopped
Black pepper to taste

TOPPING

2 tablespoons Sciabica's or
  Marsala extra virgin
  olive oil
10 whole black olives

½ teaspoon sea salt (or to
  taste)
1½ tablespoons fresh rosemary

In small mixing bowl, combine yeast with orange juice.
In large mixing bowl, add dry ingredients (flour and salt),
make well in center. Pour in yeast mixture and olive oil. Stir
to blend well. Cover and leave in warm place until doubled.
Turn out on lightly floured surface, put down, and spread
chopped olives over dough.

Knead olives; make dough into a round loaf. Place in a
lightly greased 2-quart baking pan. Lightly press in whole
olives and rosemary; drizzle top with olive oil. Let rise until
doubled in bulk. Bake covered with foil at 400° for about 30
minutes. Uncover, then bake another 15–25 minutes or until
golden brown. Makes about 1½-pound loaf. Appetizer: Slice
bread into ¼-inch-thick slices. Drizzle with olive oil; add
one or two anchovy fillets, chopped tomato, and a sprinkle
of balsamic vinegar. Add fresh basil leaves and sliced Teleme

cheese, if desired. These are best prepared as eaten rather than ahead of time.

(*Source: Cooking with California Olive Oil: Recipes from the Heart for the Heart* by Gemma Sanita Sciabica)

Stuffed Eggs

❖ ❖ ❖

6 eggs, hard cooked
2 tablespoons sweet pickled relish
4 tablespoons ham, minced (or crabmeat)
1 tablespoon cider vinegar
1 tablespoon honey
1 tablespoon prepared mustard

¼ teaspoon Tabasco sauce
Salt to taste
Pepper
Paprika to taste
Pimento-stuffed olives, for tops
2 tablespoons Marsala olive oil

Slice peeled, cooked eggs in half lengthwise; carefully scoop yolks into a bowl. Place whites on serving platter. Add relish, ham, vinegar, honey, mustard, Tabasco sauce, olive oil, salt and pepper to yolks, mash until blended. Using a spoon, fill each egg white with filling, rounding top or use a pastry bag with ½-inch star tip. Pipe filling into whites. Sprinkle stuffed eggs with paprika; place an olive slice on center of each.

Variation: *⅓ cup smoked salmon, finely chopped*

(*Source: Cooking with California Olive Oil: Recipes from the Heart for the Heart* by Gemma Sanita Sciabica)

Salads

Salads can be a great weapon in the battle against the bulge, but here's something you might not have heard: wholesome salads can be slimming as well as beautifying and anti-aging when they supply just the right nutrients.

To me, a salad often is a meal by itself. A salad should be chock-full of fresh vegetables, and fish is also an excellent ingredient. To enhance a salad and make a delicious treat, top it off with olive oil. No matter what type of olive oil you choose, you can create a wonderful slimming salad that is a complete meal or to-die-for side dish for just you or for an elegant dinner party.

These meal-sized salads are packed with all kinds of tasty, nutrient-rich ingredients, such as juicy tomatoes, flavorful feta cheese, and even black olives. Add garlic, onion, spices, and vinegar—which many of these salads contain—and you've got a heart-healthy, hearty, nutritious dish to eat solo or to share with guests for lunch or dinner.

Caesar Salad
Garden Salad with Vinaigrette
Tuna Salad Pita Pockets
Fruit Salad with Walnut Oil

Caesar Salad

❖ ❖ ❖

This classic salad calls for raw egg, so for years I've stayed clear of the potential salmonella-causing dish. I recommend hard cooking the eggs for health's sake (despite the fact as a kid we used to eat raw cake batter with eggs and I survived to tell my fur children).

½ teaspoon dry mustard
4 romaine hearts, shredded or chopped
2 garlic cloves (or to taste)
¾ cup Romano cheese, grated
2 eggs boiled 1 minute (or hard cooked)
⅓ cup Marsala olive oil
2 teaspoons Worcestershire sauce

2 tablespoons apple cider vinegar
2 tablespoons lemon or lime juice
Salt and pepper to taste
2 cups croutons made from French or Italian bread
6 anchovy filets, rinsed
½ cup radishes, sliced thin

Slice bread ½ inch thick; toast. Drizzle with olive oil; cut into cubes. Sprinkle a little cheese. In jar of blender, add olive oil, anchovies, mustard, lemon, vinegar, garlic, and Worcestershire sauce; blend. In shallow salad bowl, add romaine lettuce; scoop soft cooked eggs onto greens. Sprinkle with remaining cheese, salt, and pepper. Pour dressing over top; add croutons and radishes.

(*Source: Cooking with California Olive Oil: Recipes from the Heart for the Heart* by Gemma Sanita Sciabica)

Garden Salad with Vinaigrette

❖ ❖ ❖

A garden salad, like this one, drizzled with homemade vinaigrette is worth the time and effort to make rather than using bottled dressing or buying a premade salad. Sure, you can buy ready-made salads at the grocery store or indulge at a restaurant, but DIY salads and dressings served in the home is my cup of tea. Munching on fresh, warm, whole grain bread with a bit of olive oil is healthy and bliss.

2 cups Spring Mix (mix of baby lettuces, greens, and radicchio)
½ cup mushrooms, chopped
¼ cup green bell pepper, chopped
½ cup tomatoes, diced
2 eggs, hard boiled, sliced

¼ cup roasted sunflower seeds
½ cup cheese, shredded
1 tablespoon basil olive oil or hemp oil
1 tablespoon lemon-flavored olive oil

In a bowl, toss Spring Mix with mushrooms, bell pepper, and tomatoes. Top with eggs, seeds, cheese, and oils.

VINAIGRETTE

½ cup olive oil
3–4 tablespoons red wine vinegar

½ teaspoon mustard
Dash of freshly ground pepper

Mix oil, vinegar, mustard, and pepper. Stir before putting on salad.

Serve salad with warm French bread or whole grain rolls dipped in garlic-flavored olive oil.

Tuna Salad Pita Pockets

❖ ❖ ❖

*1 6-ounce can albacore
tuna packed in water,
drained*

*¼ cup green or red bell
pepper, chopped*

*½ cup cheese (feta or
mozzarella)*

*2 teaspoons red onion,
chopped*

*2 whole wheat pita breads,
halved, pockets opened*

*1 cup spinach lettuce,
chopped*

*2 teaspoons red wine vine-
gar*

½ cup apples, chopped

*1 teaspoon lemon-flavored
olive oil*

½ cup celery, chopped

Combine tuna with cheese and place in pita pockets.
Warm up in microwave. In a bowl, combine fruit, vegetable
mixture, and lettuce. Add vinegar and olive oil; toss. Stuff
mixture in each pita pocket half. Place pita halves on plate.
Serves 2.

Fruit Salad with Walnut Oil

❖ ❖ ❖

Back in my student era, three days a week, I commuted
from the Santa Cruz Mountains to San Francisco State
University. It was a trek. I'd go to this quaint coffee shop
complete with plants, muffins, and herbal teas. One morning I ordered plain yogurt with chunks of fresh fruit drizzled with honey. These days, I like to enhance fruit salad

with Greek yogurt, nuts, and olive oil for crunch and extra healthful flavor.

This fresh fruit salad with creamy yogurt is naturally sweet, healthy, and boasts a touch of class. Apples are usually priced right, but Honeycrisp are seasonal, a bit pricey yet worth every penny. I use orange blossom honey for the citrus punch.

3 apples, cored and diced (Honeycrisp or Fuji)	*2 tablespoons honey*
1 orange, sliced, chopped	*½ teaspoon nutmeg*
2 pears, cored and diced	*¼ cup fresh squeezed orange juice*
¼ cup dried plums or cran-berries, chopped	*1 tablespoon walnut oil*
¼ cup walnuts, chopped	*Dark chocolate shavings*
½ teaspoon cinnamon	*Greek yogurt (any flavor)*

In a large stainless-steel bowl, toss the apples, orange, pears, and plums or cranberries. Add the nuts, cinnamon, nutmeg, juice, and oil. Transfer to a glass bowl with a lid and chill in the refrigerator for 1 hour. Serve fruit salad on top of yogurt. Drizzle with olive oil and honey. Garnish with chocolate shavings. Serves 4–6.

Vegetables and Vegetarian Dishes

At 18, I became a vegetarian. I admit this announcement did not make my mother happy. She made superb dishes—all types of cuisine—from breaded veal to beef stew from scratch. But after my mom visited Europe, our meals were often more creative and daring. Think snails and squid.

I don't know if it was nutritionist Adelle Davis or the popularity of health food stores that influenced me. Perhaps it was both. I do know, however, that eating fresh vegetables, fruits, grains, yogurt, and nuts has worked to keep me—a 5-foot-5-inch woman—at 120 pounds and size 4–6 for decades.

During the gathering of these Mediterranean recipes, I learned that I can make my diet much tastier and more healthful by adding fresh onions, garlic, spices, and olive oil—especially flavored oils. The European flair is exciting to enjoy at home, especially if you can't whisk off to Italy, Spain, or Greece.

Broccoli Peanut Oil Stir-fry
Mashed Sweet Potatoes
Pizza Baguettes with Garlic Oil
Sesame-Almond Vegetable Sauté

Broccoli Peanut Oil Stir-fry

❖ ❖ ❖

Any season of the year, this flavorful stir-fry dish makes its way to my kitchen table. The vegetables, onion, garlic, honey, and rice (brown for an immunity boost) are rich in disease-fighting vitamins and minerals, exactly what the body and spirit need, and it stays true to the Mediterranean diet.

2 cups broccoli stir-fry veg-
etables (broccoli, snow
peas, carrots)
⅛ cup yellow onion, diced
1 clove garlic, crushed
1 tablespoon extra virgin
olive oil

2 teaspoons peanut oil (or,
if you prefer, rice bran
oil)
1½ cups cooked wild rice
(or brown) or quinoa
2 tablespoon pecans,
chopped

Combine onion, garlic, and vegetables in a skillet. Stir-fry in olive oil and peanut oil for a few minutes until tender but crisp. On a plate, top rice with stir-fry vegetables. Sprinkle with nuts. Serves 2–3.

The rice and vegetables are enough for a light meal. To make it extra special, I team it with store-bought deli egg rolls, drizzled with my own extra virgin olive oil and orange blossom honey. Also, hot black tea (another immune booster) is the perfect beverage with this meal. And for dessert all-natural vanilla almond or green tea ice cream with fresh berries. This vegetable and rice dish boasts layers of color (green and orange), flavors (sweet and savory), and textures (smooth and crunchy). The presentation served on white plates has a taste of exotic elegance—and switching healing oils (such as sesame oil or hemp oil) can give it a new twist, each and every time.

Mashed Sweet Potatoes

❖ ❖ ❖

*4 large sweet potatoes
(about 5 pounds), peeled
and quartered
Extra light olive oil for
greasing casserole
¼ cup extra light olive oil
1 medium onion, chopped
2–3 teaspoons grated fresh
gingerroot
¼ cup pure maple syrup
1 egg*

*2 tablespoons grated orange
peel (about 2 oranges)
1 teaspoon cinnamon
1 teaspoon salt
½ teaspoon cardamom, op-
tional
⅛ teaspoon cayenne pepper
2 slices cinnamon bread,
torn into 1-inch pieces
2 teaspoons extra light olive
oil*

Place the potatoes in a Dutch oven with enough water to
cover. Bring to a boil. Reduce the heat to medium-low, cover
loosely, and simmer 15–25 minutes or until tender.* Drain
well in a colander, place in a large bowl, and set aside.

Heat oven to 350°. Lightly oil a 2-quart casserole with
olive oil. In a medium skillet or saucepan, heat the ¼-cup
olive oil over medium heat. Add the onion and gingerroot;
cook and stir until tender.

Lightly mash the potatoes with a spoon or potato masher.
Add the onion mixture and remaining ingredients except for
the cinnamon bread and 2 teaspoons olive oil. For a smoother
consistency, beat with a mixer to blend. For a chunkier mix-

---

* Potatoes are tender when a knife can easily be inserted into the thickest
parts with little or no resistance. For a smoother casserole, cook the potatoes until very tender. For a slightly chunkier casserole, cook the potatoes
just until the knife can be inserted.

ture, mash with a potato masher or wooden spoon to blend. Spoon into the prepared casserole.

In a food processor or blender, process the bread pieces until completely chopped. Blend in the remaining 2 teaspoons of olive oil. Sprinkle over the potato mixture. Bake 35–45 minutes, or until lightly browned and thoroughly hot. Serves 18–20.

(*Source:* North American Olive Oil Association)

Pizza Baguettes with Garlic Oil

❖ ❖ ❖

12-inch store-bought whole wheat pizza crust or baguettes
¾ cup marinara sauce (with basil and olive oil)
½ cup Italian cheese, shredded
2 slices provolone cheese, shredded
2 large Roma tomatoes, chopped

1 cup fresh spinach, chopped
½ cup fresh mushrooms, chopped
¼ cup green bell pepper, chopped
1 teaspoon Herbs de Provence*
1 tablespoon garlic oil

Spread pizza crust with garlic oil. Spread crust with marinara sauce. Top with tomatoes, vegetables, cheese, spice mixture, and oil. Bake on a shallow pan at 450° for about 10 minutes, until cheese is melted and bubbly and crust is golden brown. Serves 2–4.

---

*A blend of basil, fennel, marjoram, rosemary, thyme, and a hint of lavender

Sesame-Almond Vegetable Sauté

❖ ❖ ❖

½ small (about 2 pounds) butternut or buttercup squash, peeled, seeded, and cut into ¾-inch pieces (2 cups)

1 cup baby carrots

⅓ cup chicken broth or water

1½ cups cauliflower florets (aboutt 1½ inches long)

2 cups broccoli florets (about 1½ inches long)

⅓ cup slivered almonds

¼ cup extra virgin olive oil

1 medium onion, cut into thin wedges

1 clove garlic, minced

2–3 teaspoons fresh thyme leaves

½ teaspoon salt

¼ teaspoon red pepper flakes

1 tablespoon toasted sesame seeds

In a Dutch oven or large skillet, combine the squash, carrots, and chicken broth. Cook over medium-high heat until the broth is steaming. Cover and cook 3 minutes. Add the cauliflower and broccoli; cover and cook 2–3 minutes longer, or just until the squash is tender and the broccoli is brightened. Drain and set aside.

In a small skillet over medium-high heat, cook the almonds 5–7 minutes, or until lightly golden brown, stirring frequently. Remove from the heat.

In a very large skillet or Dutch oven, heat the olive oil over medium heat. Add the onion and garlic; cook and stir 2–3 minutes, or until the onion is softened. Increase the heat to medium-high. Add the well-drained vegetable mixture, thyme, salt, and red pepper flakes. Cook and stir until hot and tender. Stir in the almonds and turn into a serving dish. Sprinkle with the sesame seeds. Serves 12.

(*Source:* North American Olive Oil Association)

Pasta

Hot pasta paired with fresh herbs and fresh French bread dipped in warm olive oil are popular combinations in the Mediterranean diet. Pasta with an assortment of vegetables, fish, garlic, onions, and olive oil is not only a scrumptious delight, but it is a healthful meal.

Think whole wheat pasta (its fiber content is higher). It's low in fat and sodium, and has 180 calories per $3/4$ cup. Also, while this type of pasta is whole grain and has no preservatives, it's also free of trans fat and cholesterol. Plus, it contains iron, riboflavin, folic acid, thiamin, and niacin. What's more, I have learned to ignore store-bought pasta sauce (its sodium content is off the charts) and replace it with fresh tomatoes. (I did find one that contains olive oil and boasts of less sodium.)

One nutritionist zapped sodium from his daily diet to lower his blood-pressure numbers. He told me that he makes his own low-sodium sauce with potassium-rich tomato paste—which makes sense, especially if you whip up a large batch and freeze it in several containers. If you, too, switch to whole wheat pasta and fresh vegetables, and add olive oil and homemade tomato paste–based sauces to your pastas, you'll come closer to a traditional Mediterranean diet, which can lead you on the path to better heart health and a longer life.

P.S.: Join me and toss out that margarine that was popular back when butter got a bad rap in the twentieth century and early twenty-first century. You can learn to dip your bread in olive oil (or other healing oils in the twenty-first century)—a European custom that is practiced in Italian restaurants from Lake Tahoe to Tuscany and in homes around the world.

Garlic Oil Fettuccini Alfredo
Spinach Pasta with Truffle Oil
Stir-fry Shrimp Linguini

Garlic Oil Fettuccine Alfredo

❖ ❖ ❖

After graduate school, I was a green journalist living on the edge. I snagged a part-time job helping a woman renovate a Victorian home in San Francisco. There was a lot of work to do, from painting, refinishing wooden floors to washing windows and clean-up chores. The work lasted for weeks—and I put my heart and soul into it. Then, one night my boss whipped up an end-of-project dinner for me. It was fettuccine—bland and boring. It didn't take a rocket scientist to figure out that she hadn't put TLC into my favorite dish, nor were there any Italian side dishes to go with the nondescript pasta. I was let down. My hard work was done, and the quickie meal was an afterthought.

I reworked the dish, but I created it with passion. I didn't cut corners. I used the best ingredients: whole grain pasta, real European-style butter, olive oils, and fresh herbs. And I didn't skimp on salad or bread. This is the thank-you meal that I would have prepared for someone's hard work for me. This meal is easy to prepare, rich, and will titillate your taste buds as if you were whisked away to a Mediterranean bistro, especially if you use olive oils and good cheeses, not just one.

12–16 ounces (cooked)
fettuccine, whole grain
1 tablespoon extra virgin
olive oil
1 tablespoon European-
style butter
½ cup 2 percent reduced-fat
organic milk
1 tablespoon garlic olive oil

½ cup half-and-half organic
milk
Fresh basil to taste
1 cup reduced-fat four-
cheese Italian cheeses
Ground pepper to taste
¼ cup goat cheese with
herbs, crumbled

In a saucepan, boil water and cook pasta until al dente. While cooking, in another pan, combine 2 percent milk, half-and-half, Italian cheeses, olive oil, garlic olive oil, and butter. On medium heat, cook until melted and a creamy sauce. Drain pasta and place in rustic baking dish. Add sauce, toss in goat cheese with herbs, basil, and pepper. Serves 4. Pair the pasta with a tossed green salad and bread teamed with olive oil. (See Appetizers and Breads section.)

Spinach Pasta with Truffle Oil

❖ ❖ ❖

8-ounce package of spinach
pasta (any shape)
3 tablespoons extra virgin
olive oil
1 tablespoon garlic olive oil
½ cup Parmesan cheese
2 garlic cloves, chopped

1 teaspoon truffle oil for
drizzling
2 cups cruciferous vegetables, chopped
Ground black pepper to
taste

In a medium pan, cook pasta per directions; drain. In a large skillet, heat extra virgin olive oil; add garlic olive oil and vegetables. Sauté until tender and fold into pasta. Toss in cheese and truffle oil. Makes 4–6 servings. Pair with fresh, warm, whole grain bread dipped in extra virgin olive oil or basil-flavored olive oil.

Stir-fry Shrimp Linguini

❖ ❖ ❖

Throughout the years, I have rebelled and gone through an anti-cooking and -baking stage. I recall one day I stocked up on those frozen pasta dinners. I'm talking mac-and-cheese to clam linguini. My freezer was stuffed with quickie microwave pasta meals for the winter. Then, in the mountains, where I befriended my saucepan and sauté pan, the aroma of onion, garlic, and spices sizzling in oil changed me and took me back to my roots as a little girl who loved to cook.

8-ounce package whole-grain linguini
1 tablespoon extra virgin olive oil
1 tablespoon butter
1 tablespoon sesame oil
¼ cup red onion, chopped
¼ cup green bell pepper, chopped

¼ cup zucchini, chopped
¼ cup Roma tomatoes, sliced
12 ounces jumbo shrimp, cooked, rinsed
½ cup fresh Parmesan cheese, shavings
Rosemary olive oil for drizzling

In a saucepan, cook pasta in boiling water until al dente. While pasta is cooking, heat olive oil and sesame oil in large sauté pan or wok over medium-high heat. Add onion, bell pepper, followed by zucchini and tomatoes. After a few minutes, add shrimp. Stir-fry until all ingredients are hot, vegetables tender. Cook for no longer than 5 minutes. Drain pasta. In a large dish, place pasta, fold in vegetables. Top with cheese. Drizzle with olive oil. Serves 4.

Poultry

Poultry, such as chicken and turkey, is included in the traditional Mediterranean diet pyramid. These days, on rare occasions, I will celebrate a holiday such as Thanskgiving and purchase an organic turkey. There are healthful benefits (lean cuts of poultry boast protein and can fill you up, not out) to having a bird in the house. And, of course, if you have a cat and two bird dogs, they will be in heaven. (No bones to the pets, please.)

Not only can you cook it up with fresh herbs, onion, and olive oil, but you can make a healthful turkey soup. I did just that last Thanksgiving and was truly thankful. I had soup to freeze, and each time I took out a container of it, I could add plenty of fresh vegetables (and olive oil) to flavor it, with no worries about the high sodium content found in store-bought soups.

Chicken Pot Pie
Cornish Game Hens with Orange Oil
Herbed Roast Turkey
Lemon-Orange Baked Chicken

Chicken Pot Pie

❖ ❖ ❖

*1 pie crust (use olive oil pie
    crust recipe, in Chapter
    9, "Combining Olive Oil
    and Vinegar" or a store-
    bought crust)*
*2½ cups chicken or turkey,
    cooked, diced*
*1 cup onions, pearl,
    blanched, peeled*
1 cup celery, sliced
1 bell pepper, chopped
1 cup mushrooms, sliced
*½ cup basil, parsley or
    mint, chopped*
*Salt, pepper, and cayenne to
    taste*

*2 carrots, cut into ½-inch
    slices*
1 potato, diced
*1 cup peas, fresh or frozen
    (or asparagus)*
½ teaspoon Tabasco
*1 cup green beans, cut into
    1-inch pieces (or sugar
    snap peas)*
¼ cup Marsala olive oil
¼ cup flour
1½ cups milk or broth
*4 garlic cloves (or to taste),
    chopped*

In saucepan, add olive oil, onions, garlic, celery, carrots,
bell peppers, and potato. Cook over medium heat until crisp
tender. Stir in flour; cook, stirring until blended. Add milk
and stir. Add remaining ingredients: peas, Tabasco, and beans.
Cook on low heat for several minutes. Pour mixture into a
greased casserole dish. Moisten rim of casserole dish with
water. Roll out pie crust, place over mixture, and press
against rim to seal. Flute edge, cut three 1-inch slits in pastry
for steam to escape while pie bakes. Brush with egg wash.
Bake at 350° for 20–25 minutes or until crust is golden brown.
Cover with foil loosely if browning too quickly.

Egg Wash

1 egg yolk beaten with 2 tablespoons water

Variation

½ cup olives
*1½ cups tomatoes,
chopped*
*Substitute beef, pork, or
meat of your choice for
chicken*

*Substitute rice, cooked, for
potatoes*
*Substitute evaporated milk
for milk*
*Pheasant, cut into bite-size
pieces*

Variation for Crust

Cut out crust into 2-inch circles; place them overlapping on top of filling; brush with egg wash. For lattice crust, cut pastry into 1-inch strips; weave over filling; brush with egg wash.

Variation for Topping

*½ cup cheddar cheese,
shredded*
*¼ cup pecans, almonds, or
nuts of your choice,
ground*

*2 tablespoons poppy or
anise seeds*
¼ cup cornmeal

(*Source: Cooking with California Olive Oil: Popular Recipes* by Gemma Sanita Sciabica)

Cornish Game Hens with Orange Oil

❖ ❖ ❖

While I traveled about America in the seventies, I don't think it occurred to me to cook game at home until the eighties, when a "kitchen" and nonvegetarian "man" were in my vocabulary. On special occasions, I do enjoy savory, protein-rich poultry, which fit in both the Mediterranean diet and the caveman-type Paleo diet foods.

2 tablespoons European-
    style butter
2 premium all-natural
    Cornish hens
2 tablespoons raw honey

⅛ cup orange-flavored olive
    oil
Ground pepper (to taste)
Fresh ginger (to taste)

In a saucepan, melt butter, honey, and oil. Wash hens and place in baking dish. Season hens. Bake for 1½ hours or until cooked. Baste periodically with honey-oil butter. Cover with foil the last 10–15 minutes. (Use a meat thermometer and when it reads 180°, it's done.) Add cooked wild rice. Serves 4.

Herbed Roast Turkey

❖ ❖ ❖

16–18-pound turkey,
    thawed if frozen
1 medium onion, cut into
    wedges

2 ribs celery, cut into 2-inch
    pieces
2 medium carrots, cut into
    2-inch pieces

4–5 stems each of fresh
sage, rosemary, and
thyme, if desired
3 cloves garlic
⅓ cup chopped fresh sage
leaves
¼ cup fresh rosemary
leaves

3 tablespoons fresh thyme
leaves
½ teaspoon salt
½ teaspoon pepper
⅓ plus ½ cup virgin olive
oil

Heat oven to 325°. Remove the giblets and neck from the turkey; discard or save for broth, if desired. Rinse the cavity of the turkey and pat dry. Sprinkle the inside of the turkey with salt and pepper. Place the onion, celery, carrot, and, if desired, 1–2 stems each of the sage, rosemary, and thyme inside the turkey. Place the turkey on a rack in a roasting pan; set aside.

In a food processor or blender, chop the garlic until fine. Add the herb leaves; pulse until coarsely chopped. Add the salt and pepper. With the machine running, add the ⅓ cup olive oil and process until well blended.

Carefully separate (but do not remove) the skin from the meat on the breast of the turkey. Rub 2 tablespoons of the herb mixture between the meat and skin. Replace the skin. If desired, add 1 cup water or broth to the pan under the rack. Roast the turkey 1 hour.

Meanwhile, blend the remaining ½ cup olive oil into the remaining herb mixture. If desired, bundle the remaining herb stems together to form a "basting brush." After 1 hour of roasting, baste the turkey with part of the herb mixture.

Continue roasting the turkey 2½–3¼ hours* or until the

---

*The total roasting time will be about 12–20 minutes per pound, depending on the size of the turkey. Check the turkey wrapper for additional timing information. This olive oil–herb mixture can also be used when roasting only a turkey breast, and is also excellent on roasted or grilled chicken or pork.

internal temperature of the thickest part of the thigh is 170°
and the juice runs clear, basting every hour. If necessary,
cover the breast of the turkey with foil to prevent overbrowning during roasting. Remove from oven and let stand
10–15 minutes before carving. Serves 16–20.

(*Source:* North American Olive Oil Association)

Lemon-Orange Baked Chicken

❖ ❖ ❖

In the twenty-first-century, I can't imagine making fried
chicken. Occasionally, for a special holiday, I'll go for baked
since poultry is included in the traditional Mediterranean
diet. Instead of using gooey Crisco (like my mom did back in
the twentieth century), olive oil is the dietary fat of choice.

2 chicken breasts, skinned and deboned	*1 tablespoon lemon juice, fresh*
2 tablespoons extra virgin olive oil	*1 tablespoon blood orange olive oil*
Ground black pepper	*2 tablespoons orange blossom honey*
½ teaspoon Mediterranean sea salt	

Preheat oven to 375°. Rinse chicken and dry. Place in
baking dish. Drizzle extra virgin olive oil on top. Sprinkle
with pepper and salt. Top with lemon juice. Bake for approximately 40 minutes or until brown and crispy. Glaze with
mixture of orange olive oil and honey.

Bake for another few minutes. Serves 2.

Fish

While I prefer to be a strict vegetarian, it's a challenge to do it right and maintain good health. I know that I need essential fatty acids for good health. So, two to three times per week, I try to include fresh salmon or tuna in my diet. In my early teens, I do recall indulging in lobster, trout, halibut, shrimp, and scallops.

I recall a meal at Cannery Row in Monterey, California. It was the first time that I had the Cioppino experience—fun, and it is for the uninhibited fish lover. Mediterranean people do eat and love fresh, grilled fish. And, fish does play a role in the health perks of Mediterranean diets.

Cioppino
Halibut with Caper Sauce
Simple Salmon

Cioppino

❖ ❖ ❖

¼ cup Marsala Olive Fruit Oil
1 onion, diced
6 cloves garlic, chopped
1 bell pepper, diced
¾ cup wine
4 cups chopped fresh or canned tomatoes

4 tablespoons tomato paste
Salt, pepper, and red hot pepper flakes to taste
2 bay leaves (remove before serving)
½ cup chopped fresh basil and/or parsley

½ *pound cod, cut into*
  2-inch cubes
1 pound crab (Alaskan
  King, thawed)

1 pound shrimp
2 dozen clams or mussels
½ *pound scallops*

In a Dutch oven, add the oil, onions, garlic, and bell pepper. Cook over medium heat until soft. Add the wine and cook 1 minute. Add the tomatoes, tomato paste, salt, pepper, red hot pepper flakes, and bay leaves. Simmer for 15 minutes, covered, then add the basil. Add the cod and cook for about 5 minutes. Add the remaining fish and cook, covered, for 5 minutes, or until the clams open. Discard any unopened clams. Serve in soup bowls with toasted crusty Italian bread slices.*

VARIATIONS

Flounder fillets or lobster, cubed
2 cups small potatoes, cubed
1 small head escarole, chopped
Snapper or sea bass, cubed
¼ cup pesto sauce

(*Source: Cooking with California Olive Oil: Treasured Family Recipes* by Gemma Sanita Sciabica)

*Cioppino is a favorite in San Francisco, where it is served with sourdough bread and a bib.

Halibut with Caper Sauce

❖ ❖ ❖

2 tablespoons drained and roughly chopped capers

¼ cup chopped cornichon pickles

2 hard-cooked eggs, peeled and finely diced

⅓ cup chopped Italian parsley

¼ cup The Olive Press California Mission Extra Virgin Olive Oil

1 tablespoon fresh lemon juice

Salt and pepper to taste

1 cup flour

4 halibut fillets (6–7 ounces each)

2–3 tablespoons vegetable oil

Lemon wedges

Combine the capers, cornichons, eggs, parsley, olive oil, and lemon juice in a bowl. Whisk well so that the egg yolks begin to break down and make the sauce creamier. Season with salt and pepper. Set aside.

Put the flour in a shallow bowl. Season the fish with salt and pepper, then completely dredge it in the flour. Heat 2 tablespoons vegetable oil in a skillet, then add 2 halibut fillets flesh-side down. Cook for about 5 minutes, turn the fish over, and cook another 5 minutes for medium doneness. Transfer to a warmed plate. Repeat with the other 2 fillets, adding more oil to the pan if necessary. Spoon the sauce over the fish and garnish with the lemon wedges. Serves 4.

(*Source:* The Olive Press)

Simple Salmon

❖ ❖ ❖

6 salmon filets (6 ounces
    each)
1 tomato, peeled, seeded,
    and diced
4 ounces sliced yellow
    onion
2 ounces sliced carrots
1 lemon, sliced into rounds
2 cloves garlic, sliced

8 ounces vegetable broth
2 ounces olive oil
2 ounces red wine vinegar
2 ounces dry red wine
2 bay leaves
3 fresh thyme sprigs
4 fresh tarragon leaves
Salt and pepper to taste

Place the 6 salmon filets in an oven-proof glass pan. Add
all the other ingredients. Marinate for 1 hour in the refrigerator. In the same glass pan, cover the salmon loosely with a
piece of foil and bake for 15 minutes at 350°. When the
salmon is done, remove it to a service plate. Strain the liquid
from the baking pan and reduce it to less than a cup using a
whisk. Adjust the seasonings, and pour the liquid over
salmon. Serves 6.

(Recipe created by Chef Salvatore J. Campagna)

Desserts

I remember in the film *Under the Tuscan Sun* when Katherine (Lindsay Duncan) indulges guilt-free in an ice-cream cone and Frances (Diane Lane) takes a peek at the uninhibited woman enjoying herself. It's healthier to eat your favorite foods in moderation than to deprive yourself of life's simple pleasures, which can lead to overeating. While processed cakes, cookies, and ice creams are not healthful (usually because they contain too much sugar, preservatives, and artery-clogging trans fat), homemade desserts can be good for you. Also, anytime you can pair fresh fruit with cookies or cake, by all means do as they do in Europe and pile on the best fruit of the season.

Chocolate Chip Oatmeal Cookies
Rocky Road Tea Bark
Peppermint Bark with a Citrus Twist
The Olive Press Citrus Cake

Chocolate Chip Oatmeal Cookies

❖ ❖ ❖

*⅓ cup Sciabica Orange
  Olive Oil*
1 large egg
⅓ cup sugar
⅓ cup brown sugar
1 teaspoon vanilla
*½ teaspoon Watkins Danish
  pastry extract*

¼ cup orange juice or milk
1 cup flour
*¾ cup uncooked quick-
  cooking oats*
1 teaspoon baking soda
¼ teaspoon salt
½ cup chocolate chips
¼ cup currants or raisins

Preheat oven to 375°. Spray a large cookie sheet with non-stick cooking spray. In a mixing bowl, mix the olive oil, egg, sugars, flavorings, and orange juice; stir to blend. Add the flour, oats, baking soda, and salt, and stir until combined. Fold in the chocolate chips and currants.

Drop by level tablespoons (or with a 1-inch ice-cream scooper) 2 inches apart onto Reynolds aluminum (release) foil-lined cookie sheet. Flatten slightly with water-moistened tines of fork.

Bake 12–14 minutes, or until golden brown. Cool on a wire rack. Frost as desired.

(*Source: Cooking with California Olive Oil: Treasured Family Recipes* by Gemma Sanita Sciabica)

Rocky Road Tea Bark

❖ ❖ ❖

7 ounces premium baking chips, 60 percent cacao bittersweet chocolate

7 ounces premium baking chips, milk chocolate

1 cup miniature marsh-mallows

1 tablespoon macadamia nut oil

½ cup macadamia nuts, chopped (place in plastic bag and use a hammer to crush into bite-size bits)

¼ cup tea leaves (green tea with citrus notes)

Melt dark chocolate chips in microwave for about 2–3 minutes, stirring occasionally until melted. Stir the dark chocolate and spread it onto a nonstick cookie sheet (or line with parchment paper). Spread and shape into a rectangle. Chill in freezer for about 10 minutes. Meanwhile, melt milk chocolate chips in microwave. Once the chocolate is melted, stir in nut oil; fold in marshmallows and nuts. (Save half of the nuts for the top.) Take out dark chocolate from freezer and frost with the rocky road mixture. Sprinkle with nuts and tea on top. Put back into freezer for 10 minutes. Take out and pick up the entire chocolate candy slab, then place on a plate. If you use parchment paper, take it off. Break into peanut brittle–like square pieces. Place in airtight sealed containers and keep in refrigerator.

Peppermint Bark with a Citrus Twist

❖ ❖ ❖

Ah, peppermint bark is a specialty item available during the winter holidays that can help warm the heart and beat the blues. It's a mix of red and white peppermint candy canes sprinkled on white chocolate on top of good-for-you dark chocolate. While I've enjoyed store-bought peppermint bark, the irregular, rustic, peanut-brittle–shaped home-style kind is so much sweeter.

The pieces of delicious bark can be stored in the fridge. Use small containers and give to friends and family as gifts or a self-gift. Either way, it's festive and is a feel-good treat. Peppermint bark made with superfoods dark chocolate and olive oil give me a feeling of accomplishment.

7 ounces premium baking chips, 60% cacao bitter-sweet chocolate
7 ounces premium baking chips, classic white
12 peppermint candy canes, crushed (place in plastic

bag and use a hammer to crush into bite-size bits)
1 teaspoon orange-flavored olive oil
1 teaspoon lemon-flavored olive oil

Melt dark chocolate chips in a microwave for about 2–3 minutes, stirring occasionally until melted. Stir the dark chocolate, adding orange-flavored olive oil, and spread it onto a nonstick flat cookie sheet (or line with parchment paper). Spread and shape into a rectangle. Chill in freezer for about 10 minutes. Meanwhile, melt white chocolate chips in the microwave. Once the white chocolate is melted, add lemon-flavored olive oil and stir in half of the candy-cane mixture. Take out dark chocolate from the freezer and frost with white chocolate and candy-cane mixture. Sprinkle crushed candy canes on top. Put back into freezer for 10 minutes. Take out and pick up the entire chocolate candy slab, then place on a plate. (If you use parchment paper, take it off. Break into nice sized pieces. (Or use chilled cookie cutters if preferred for perfect shapes.

The Olive Press Citrus Cake

❖ ❖ ❖

Grated zest and juice of 1 lemon
Grated zest and juice of 1 orange
⅓ cup The Olive Press Blood Orange (or The Olive Press Meyer Lemon) Olive Oil
1 cup sugar
¼ teaspoon salt

3 medium eggs
1½ cups semolina
1 cup tightly packed ground almonds
1 teaspoon almond essence
1 teaspoon baking powder
1 teaspoon orange flower water
¼ cup Cointreau or Grand Marnier

Preheat the oven to 325°. Reserve a little of the grated lemon and orange zest, and put the remainder in a bowl with the oil, sugar, salt, orange and lemon juices, and eggs. Beat together with a whisk until light and fluffy and doubled in volume.

Sieve the semolina and baking powder into a second bowl and add the ground almonds. Fold the almond essence and orange flower water into the egg mixture. Pour all at once into the dry ingredients and fold together, but do not over-mix. Spoon into a 9-inch springform pan, lightly oiled and lined with parchment, and smooth the top. Sprinkle the reserved lemon and orange zest over the top.

Bake near the top of the oven for 40–50 minutes, or until pale gold at the edges and firm in the middle. A toothpick inserted into the center should come out clean.

Remove from the oven and let cool in the pan for about 10 minutes. Drizzle the liqueur over the top. Push the cake out, still on the loose metal base, and let it cool on a wire rack for another 10 minutes. Remove the base and paper. Serve in 8–12 wedges, warm or cooled. Do not refrigerate. The cake will keep in an airtight container for up to 4 days.

(*Source:* The Olive Press)

A FINAL DISH ON OILS

Nowadays, I feel like I must look like a sturdy, growing, and aging olive tree at peace. It's true. I'm an age-defying baby boomer in my prime. So, it was my mission to revisit Olive Oil Land *and* branch out (pun intended) to experience other healing oils for the thrill and health of it, like going to an amusement park and trying different rides.

So, as I end my exciting food adventure in the world of oils and fats, part of me doesn't want to leave. After all, there are so many oils that I haven't tried—and want to dabble in for cooking and baking, much like when I wrote the books on vinegar, chocolate, honey, and coffee. The deal is, once you enter the world of superfoods, like olive oil, it's difficult to go back and use only one cooking oil—no other oils. It would be like using only orange blossom honey or the same brand of joe every day. Variety in the land of oils is the spice in creating and eating food for the body and spirit.

When I cook a casserole or stir-fry and bake cookies to muffins, I don't grab a basic nondescript vegetable oil, I now have olive oils—so many kinds—and an arsenal of other healing oils (including tropical oils and nut oils) that enhance dishes with amazing flavor and texture to live for and remember.

I am an accidental health-nut foodie, and I enjoy cooking and baking—and doing it my way. Using different olive oils and other plant-based cooking oils (plus butter from European-style to organic grass-fed milk) makes dishes more exciting. When people think of oil as something you put on your salad or toss in a dish, I shake my head, and think, *You haven't been to Olive Oil Land.* Once you take the trip, and experiment with other healing oils, too, you'll get what I mean. There is no going back to the days of lard and margarine. In the world of different oils you can find anything and everything that'll titillate your taste buds and nourish your body, mind, and soul. And this essential guide to oils will be your roadmap.

PART 8

OLIVE OIL RESOURCES

Where Can You Buy Olive Oil?

As olive oil (and other healing oils) continues to be praised for its powerful health benefits, quality olive oils for the health-conscious and specialty olive oils for olive oil enthusiasts are popping up everywhere around the globe. Currently, a wide world of oils can be bought in supermarkets, specialty stores, and health food stores, as well as through mail order and the Internet. And yes, the decision regarding which one is best can be subjective, just like when choosing your favorite dog breed. Remember, both pure, quality olive oils and canines are judged in the real world.

Here is a list of olive oils, and other types of oils, from organic and natural to commercial brands. If you're interested in buying any of these popular oils and can't find them locally, just contact the manufacturers directly for the locations of stores nearest you.

OLIVE OILS PURCHASED IN RETAIL OUTLETS

Bertolli
800-670-7356
www.villabertolli.com

Olive oils and vinegars

Lucini Italia
888-5LUCINI
www.lucini.com

Extra virgin olive oil, artesan vinegar

OLIVE OIL BEAUTY PRODUCTS

Cali Cosmetics, Inc.
101 W. 23rd Street, Suite 226
New York, NY 10011
888-883-CALI
www.calicosmetics.com

Products include "extracts of Italian olive oil," such as Moisturizing Olive Oil Soap and Cali Travel Spa, body and bath skin care, home fragrances, candles, soaps, perfumes, travel, and household items.

Olivella
888-OLIVELLA
www.olivella@usa.com

A premiere line for personal skin care made from 100% virgin olive oil. Olivella skin products are made right where the olives are grown, in the region of Umbria known as the "Green Heart of Italy." Products include Face and Body Bar, Face and Body Liquid Soap, Hand Cream, and Body Cream.

SuperCrema Skincare Italy
561-372-8020
www.supercremaskincare.com

Italy's balm for face and body made from 100% organic extra virgin olive oil, beeswax, and sweet almond oil.

OLIVE OIL MILLS AND PRODUCERS IN CALIFORNIA

Apollo Olive Oil
P.O. Box 1054
Oregon House, CA 95962
877-776-0703
www.apollooliveoil.com

Apollo Olive Oils are among the best in California. Certified both organic and extra virgin, they are also raw unadulterated and 100% cold-pressed on the vacuum mill designed in Tuscany to preserve the highest levels of flavor, nutrients, and good-for-you antioxidants.

California Olive Ranch (COR)
2675 Lone Tree Road
Oroville, CA 95965
530-846-8000

Chico Office
1367 E. Lassen Avenue, Suite A-1
Chico, CA 95973
www.californiaoliveranch.com

COR offers:

- *Arbequina Extra Virgin Olive Oil*
- *Arbosan Extra Virgin Olive Oil*
- *Estate Reserve Blend*

Frantoio Ristorante and Olive Oil Co.
152 Shoreline Highway
Mill Valley, CA 94941
415-289-5777
www.frantoio.com

Frantoio Ristorante and Olive Oil Co. is the only restaurant in the United States with an in-house, state-of-the-art olive oil production facility. At its Web site you can order its premium Certified California and Tuscan Extra Virgin Olive Oils.

Nick Sciabica & Sons
2150 Yosemite Boulevard
Modesto, CA 95354-3931
209-577-5067; 800-551-9612

Sciabicia specializes in cold-pressed olive oils, using several varieties of California olives. They also provide natural red wine vinegar, as well as balsamic vinegar imported from Modena, Italy. Sciabica offers a variety of extra virgin olive oils. Also, Sciabica's "Speciality Olive Oils" include flavored products containing basil, garlic, jalapeño, lemon, and orange.

These oils contain no artificial flavors, but are made by crushing and cold-pressing together the ingredients and fresh Mission Variety olives in the mill.

Pasolivo
8530 Vineyard Drive
Paso Robles, CA 93446
805-227-0186
www.pasolivo.com

Pasolivo olive oils are made in Paso Robles, California, on the state's central coast. They hand-pick their own olives and press them just steps away in their own olive press. The olives are grown organically and sustainably. Pasolivo offers several California Certified extra-virgins and a range of flavors, including Meyer Lemon and Rosemary.

The Olive Press
24724 Highway Arnold Drive
Hwy 121
Sonoma, CA 95476
800-965-4839
www.theolivepress.com

The Olive Press was established in 1985 as the first olive mill in Sonoma. They are dedicated to making only the finest award-winning California extra virgin olive oil in their facility that is designed to meet custom pressing needs of commercial producers, growers, and small harvests, and hobbyists wishing to create "estate" olive oil from homegrown olives. The Olive Press Tasting Room and Artisian Market as well as their online store are dedicated to olives and olive oil. They also offer balsamic vinegars and a variety of pantry items.

Round Pond
886 Rutherford Road
888-302-2575
Rutherford, CA 94573
www.roundpond.com

Searching for a Mediterranean-type escape—tours and tast-ings—with a fascinating olive mill tour and adventure of Round Pond artisanal olive oils and wine vinegars? Discover every-thing you want to know about olive cultivation, harvest, and production before indulging yourself in a guided tasting that includes locally made bread, cheese, and fresh produce.

OTHER HEALING OILS AND FATS

Kerrygold Butter
Irish Dairy Board, Inc./U.S. Office
1007 Church Street, Suite 800
Evanston, IL 60201
www.kerrygoldusa.com

Butter made from the milk of grass-fed cows. Salted Butter, Un-salted Butter, Garlic & Herb Butter, and Naturally Softer Pure Irish Butter. Available in grocery stores and more locations.

Nutiva
213 West Cutting Blvd.
Richmond, CA 94804
800-993-4367

Since 1999 they have operated an innovative company pro-viding organic superfood, including coconut oil, hemp oil, and red palm oil.

Premier Organics
810 81st Ave. #B
Oakland, CA 94621
866-237-8688

Artisanal organic raw coconut oil, extra virgin, artisanal raw coconut butter.

Tropical Traditions
888-311-2626
www.tropicaltraditions.com

Their Gold Label Virgin Coconut Oil is their highest quality coconut oil. This premium oil is hand-crafted by family producers in the Philippines using traditional methods passed down from generations. This company is one of the pioneers to export coconut oil to the U.S., back in 2001.

SPECIALTY FOODS

ChefShop.com
1425 Elliot Avenue West
Seattle, WA 98119
800-596-0885
www.ChefShop.com

ChefShop.com carries an extensive line of artisan-produced specialty foods and ingredients from around the world, including a selection of healing oils such as rice bran oil and organic black truffle oil, macadamia nut oil, organic mandarin olive oil, and other gourmet items like organic dark chocolate with olive oil bon bons. Stop by the retail store anytime for a personalized olive oil and vinegar tasting.

King Arthur Flour
The Baker's Store
135 US Rt. 5 South
Norwich, Vermont 05055
800-827-6836
www.kingarthurflour.com

Specialty items for all your cooking and baking needs, including Herbs De Provence, and garlic oil. If you have questions about the King Arthur Flour recipes in this book, call their baker's hot line at 800-649-3717.

OLIVE OIL ONLINE FROM FRANCE, ITALY, AND SPAIN

In 1996, Judy Ridgway was appointed by the Italian Mastri Oleari (Masters of Olive Oil) to sit as the first non-Italian judge on the judging panel for the prestigious Leone d'Oro Awards for olive oil. She sat on the panel each year until 2001. She provides these top-notch producers in three European regions but made it clear that it is a difficult choice. "There are so many good ones in each of these countries and all very different. Anyway, I will stick a pin in the lists," she says.

Here are several producers worth writing home about to Mediterranean cuisine lovers and anyone interested in extra virgin olive oil.

France
Castelas
www.castelas.com

Italy
Colonna
www.marinacolonna.it
Frantoio Franci
www.frantoiofranci.it

Spain
Marqués de Valdueza
www.marquesdevaldueza.com

OLIVE OIL ONLINE FROM OTHER REGIONS AROUND THE GLOBE

Olive Connexions International Pte. Ltd.
170 Upper Bukit Timah Road
#13-04
Bukit TImah Shopping Centre
Singapore 588179
www.oliveconnexions.com

OLIVE OIL LAMPS

Lehman's
289 Kurzen Road North
Dalton, OH 44618
www.lehmans.com

Lehman's carries a full line of modern lamps that burn olive oil and other vegetable oils. To order its 160-page catalog of lamps and much more, contact the company.

COFFEE TO PAIR WITH OLIVE OIL

Jelks Gourmet Coffee Roasters
P.O. Box 8667
Shreveport, LA 71148
800-235-7361
www.jelks-coffee.com

More than 200 gourmet flavored coffees that contain no sugar, no calories, and no cholesterol. Some flavors pair well with healing oils and fats, such as almond, butter pecan, coconut cream, and Hawaiian macadamia nut.

HONEY TO PAIR WITH OLIVE OIL

Honey Ridge Farms
12310 NE 245th Avenue
Brush Prairie, WA 98606
360-256-0086
www.honeyridgefarms.com

Unforgettable gourmet honey, honey crèmes (apricot, blackberry, clover, lemon, raspberry), honey vinegar, and honey grilling sauces and glazes.

OLIVE LEAF TEAS

Olivus Olive Leaf Teas Source
www.olivus.com

Olivus is a company dedicated to the benefits of the olive and its leaf, oil, and fruit. Olive leaf is available in capsule, extract, and tea form. Olive leaf tea is an organic, caffeine-free, natural source of antioxidants shown to fight bacteria and viruses, promote circulation, increase energy, and more.

ORGANIZATIONS

North American Olive Oil Association
3301 Route 66, Suite 205, Bldg. C
Neptune, NJ 07753
732-922-3008
www.naooa.org

This association is committed to: supplying North America consumers with quality products in a fair and competitive environment; providing an understanding of the various grades of olive oil; and informing about the benefits of liquid gold in nutrition, health, and the culinary arts. The International Olive Council is a quasi–United Nations organization.

INFORMATION ON OLIVE OIL

California Olive Oil Council (COOC)
801 Camelia Street, Suite D
Berkeley, CA 94707
888-718-9830
www.cooc.com

Looking for past or current news, health questions, and events? You will find it all from this organization established in 1992. The mission of the COOC is to promote the fresh, quality extra virgin olive oils made in California. Through its Seal Certification program, it helps everyone from chefs to restaurants find guaranteed extra virgin olive oils for their kitchens. Its membership also welcomes consumers and olive oil producers.

International Olive Oil Council (IOOC)
Principe de Vergara 154
28002 Madrid, Spain
www.internationaloliveoil.org

The IOOC is a UN-chartered body that regulates olive oil throughout most of the world, but not in the United States.

The Olive Oil Source
www.oliveoilsource.com

A newsletter with a wealth of information about U.S. olive oil companies, international growers, olive oil sales, health, recipes, and much more.

OLIVE OIL MUSEUMS

Adatepe Olive Oil Museum
www.adatepe.com/en

Museo dell' Olivo
www.museodellolivo.com

Inaugurated in 1992, the Olive Tree Museum receives more than 30,000 visitors annually. The Olive Tree Museum is an Italian private museum, created to portray the olive tree, symbolic of the Mediterranean.

ADDITIONAL INFORMATION

Experience the Olive Harvest
Umbria, Provincia di Perugia, Italy
www.rogaia.com

Villa La Rogaia is an organic farm that cultivates olive trees, produces the finest extra virgin olive oil, and raises medicinal herbs and fragrant plants. Adopt an olive tree at La Rogaia and get olive oil from your own tree. Or come to La Rogaia for a holiday in November and experience the olive harvest, picking your own olive oil.

As of this writing, I find that more manufacturers and retail outlets could be added to this list. However, because of the surge of interest in olive oil and the varied types of oil to choose from, it is impossible to keep up with all the new companies marketing such products. A wide world of olive oil awaits you and your own personal experiences.

Notes

CHAPTER 1:
THE POWER OF OLIVE OIL

1. "Olive Quotes," Food Reference website, www.food reference.com /html/qolives.html (accessed July 13, 2007).
2. "What Experts Say," The Olive Tree World, www.olivetree. eat-online.net/framehealth.htm (accessed July 13, 2007).
3. Ibid.
4. Liz Applegate, *101 Miracle Foods That Heal Your Heart* (Paramus, NJ: Prentice-Hall Press, 2000), p. 194.

CHAPTER 2:
A GENESIS OF THE OLIVE

1. "Olive Tree Quotes," Food Reference website, www. foodreference. com/html/qolivetrees.html (accessed July 13, 2007).
2. "Rossdhu Olive Oils—Health and Olive Oil," Rossdhu, www.colquhounolives.com.au/health.html (accessed July 13, 2007).
3. David Stewart, *Healing Oils of the Bible* (Marble Hill, MO: Care Publications, 2003), p. 97.
4. Ibid., p. 155.
5. "Olive Oil Facts," Pukara Estate, www.pukaraestate. com.au/Content_Common/pg-Olive-Oil-Facts.seo (accessed July 13, 2007).

6. Ibid.
7. Ibid.
8. Ibid.
9. "The 6,000 Year History of Olive Oil," Filippo Berio, www.filippoberio.com/Tradition/History.asp (accessed July 13, 2007).
10. "Olive Oil Facts," Pukara Estate, www.pukaraestate.com.au/Content Common/pg-Olive-Oil-Facts.seo (accessed July 13, 2007).
11. "The 6,000 Year History of Olive Oil," Filippo Berio, www.filippoberio.com/Tradition/History.asp (accessed July 13, 2007).
12. "Olive Oil," United Nations Conference on Trade and Development, www.unctad.org/infocom/anglais/olive/characteristics.htm (accessed July 13, 2007).
13. "The Olive Tree and Olive Oil in Crete and Greece," Explore Crete, www.explorecrete.com/nature/olive.html (accessed July 13, 2007).

CHAPTER 3:
A HISTORICAL TESTIMONY

1. "The Greek Romance with the Olive," The Hindu Business Line, www.thehindubusinessline.com (accessed July 13, 2007).
2. Charles Quest-Ritson, *Olive Oil* (New York: DK Publishing, 2006), p. 252.

CHAPTER 4:
WHERE ARE THE SECRET INGREDIENTS?

1. "Pleasures of the Table Quotes," Food Reference website, www.foodreference.com/html/qoliveoil.html (accessed July 13, 2007).

CHAPTER 5:
WHY IS OLIVE OIL SO HEALTHY?

1. David Stewart, *Healing Oils of the Bible* (Marble Hill, MO: Care Publications, 2003), p. 159.
2. M. Covas, *Annals of Internal Medicine*, 145 (September 5, 2006), pp. 333–341.
3. David Stewart, *Healing Oils of the Bible* (Marble Hill, MO: Care Publications, 2003), p. 159.
4. Erin L. Richman, et al., "Fat Intake After Diagnosis and Risk of Lethal Prostate Cancer and All-Cause Mortality." *JAMA Intern Med.* 2013. 1 DOI: 10-1001/jamainternmed.20133.6536.
5. "Effects of Olive Oils in Biomarkers of Oxidative DNA Stress in Northern and Southern Europeans," *The Federation of American Societies for Experimental Biology Journal,* 21 (2007): pp. 45–52.
6. JA Menendez, L Vellon, R Colomer, and R Lupu, "Oleic Acid, the Main Monounsaturated Fatty Acid of Olive Oil, Suppresses Her-2/neu (erbB-2) Expression and Synergistically Enhances the Growth Inhibitory Effects of Trastuzumab (HerceptinTM) in Breast," *Annals of Oncology* (January 10, 2005). "Prevention of Diabetes with Mediterranean Diets."
7. Salvadó-Salas Jordi, M.D., Ph.D., et al., *Ann Intern Med.* 2014; 160 (1):1-10-10.

8. David Stewart, *Healing Oils of the Bible* (Marble Hill, MO: Care Publications, 2003), p. 162.

9. Nikolaos Scarmeas et al., "Mediterranean Diet, Alzheimer Disease, and Vascular Mediation," *Archives of Neurology*, 63 (2006): pp. 1709–77.

10. Martinez, H.-Lapiscina, Elena, *J Neurol Neurosurg Psychiatry doi:* 10:1136. "Mediterranean Diet Improves Cognition: The PREMED-NAVARRA Randomized Trial," published online first, 13 May 2013.

CHAPTER 6:
THE KEYS TO THE MEDITERRANEAN DIET

1. "Food Quotes," ThinkExist.com, www.thinkexist.com/quotations/food (accessed July 13, 2007).

2. "The World Health Report 2006," World Health Organization, www.who.int/countries/en (accessed July 13, 2007).

3. *The Journal of the American Medical Association,* February 8, 2006.

4. *The New England Journal of Medicine*, "Primary Prevention of Cardiovascular Disease with a Mediterranean Diet; published Feb. 25, 2012 at NEJM.org.

5. Samieri, Cecilia, Ph.D., et al., *Ann Intern Med.* 2013; 1 159 (9): 584–591. "The Association Between Dietary Patterns at Midlife and Health in Aging: An Observational Study."

CHAPTER 7:
FLAVORED OLIVE OILS

1. "Perfection Quotes," Food Reference website, www.foodreference.com/html/qperfection.html (accessed July 13, 2007).
2. Michael Chiarello, *Flavored Oils and Vinegars: 100 Recipes for Cooking with Infused Oils and Vinegars* (San Francisco: Chronicle Books, 2006), p. 85.
3. Ibid., p. 85.

CHAPTER 8:
MORE HEALING OILS

1. "What Experts Say," The Olive Tree World, www.olivetree.eat-online.net/framehealth.htm (accessed July 13, 2007).
2. American Heart Association's EPI/NPAM 2013 Scientific Session in New Orleans.
3. Mary G. Enig, "Flaxseed and Flaxseed Oils for Omega-3 Fatty Acids," The Weston A. Price Foundation for Wise Traditions, www.westonaprice.org/knowyourfats/flaxseed.html (accessed July 13, 2007).
4. Malhotra, Aseem, et al., "Saturated Fat Is Not the Major Issue," *BMJ* 2013; 347:f6340.

CHAPTER 9:
COMBINING OLIVE OIL AND VINEGAR

1. "Aeschylus," Bartleby.com, www.bartleby.com/66/45/3045.html (accessed July 13, 2007).

2. Jim Long, "Dress for Success," The Herb Companion, www.herb companion.com (accessed July 13, 2007).

CHAPTER 10:
THE ELIXIR TO HEART HEALTH

1. "What Experts Say," The Olive Tree World, www.olivetree.eat-online.net/framehealth.htm (accessed July 13, 2007).
2. Steven Pratt and Kathy Matthews, *SuperFoods Rx: Fourteen Foods That Will Change Your Life* (New York: William Morrow, 2004), p. 112.
3. Editors of FC&A Medical Publishing, *The Folk Remedy Encyclopedia: Olive Oil, Vinegar, Honey and 1,001 Other Home Remedies* (Peachtree City, GA: FC&A Medical Publishing, 2001), p. 168.
4. Ibid.
5. K. Covas, HE. Nyyssonen, et al., "The Effect of Polyphenols in Olive Oil on Heart Disease Risk Factors," *Annals of Internal Medicine 145* (2006): pp. 333–341.
6. Katherine Esposito et al., "Effect of a Mediterranean-Style Diet on Endothelial Dysfunction and Markers of Vascular Inflammation in the Metabolica Syndrome," *Journal of the American Medical Association,* 292 (September 22–29, 2004): pp. 1440–1446.

CHAPTER 11:
THE OLIVE OIL DIET

1. "What Experts Say," The Olive Tree World, www.olivetree.eat-online.net/framehealth.htm (accessed July 13, 2007).
2. P. Schieberle, "Identifiying substances that regulate satiety in oils and fat foodstuffs by adding lipid compounds with high satiety effect; finding of the DFG/AiF cluster project 'Perception of fat content and regulating satiety: an approach to developing low-fat foodstuffs.'" 2009–2012.
3. Frank Sabino, et al., "Olive oil aroma extract modulates cerebral blood flow in gustatory brain areas in humans," *AmjClinNutr,* November 2013, vol. 98, no. 5, 1360–1366.
4. Seth Roberts, *The Shangri-La Diet: The No Hunger Eat Anything Weight-Loss Plan* (New York: Putnam, 2006), p. 30.
5. Ibid., p. 31.

CHAPTER 12:
ANTIAGING WONDER FOOD

1. "Olive Oil Quotes," Food Reference website, www.foodreference.com/html/qoliveoil.html (accessed July 13, 2007).
2. Extra virgin olive oil consumption and antioxidant status in healthy institutionalized elderly humans published in *Archives of Gerontology and Geriatrics*, Volume 57, Issue 2, September– October 2013, pages 234–242. Maria-Jesús Oliveras-López.

CHAPTER 13:
CURES FROM YOUR KITCHEN

1. "The Olive Tree and Olive Oil in Crete and Greece," Explore Crete, www.explorecrete.com/nature/olive.html (accessed July 13, 2007).

CHAPTER 14:
OLIVE OIL MANIA: USING OLIVE OIL FOR THE HOUSEHOLD, KIDS, PETS, AND BEAUTY

1. "Hemingway, Ernest," Bartleby.com, www.bartleby.com (accessed July 13, 2007).
2. Carol Firenze, *The Passionate Olive: 101 Things to Do with Olive Oil* (New York: Ballantine Books, 2005), p. 144.
3. Ibid., p. 148.
4. Ibid., p. 145.

CHAPTER 15:
OLIVE BEAUTIFUL

1. "Olive Branch Quotes," ThinkExist.com, www.think exist.com/quotations/food (accessed July 13, 2007).

CHAPTER 16:
OLIVE OIL PRODUCERS, TASTING BARS, AND TOURS

1. "Olive Oil Quotes," Food Reference website, www.food

references.com/html/qoliveoil.html (accessed July 13, 2007).

2. Charles Quest-Ritson, *Olive Oil* (New York: DK Publishing, 2006), p. 135.
3. Ibid, p. 53.
4. Ibid, p. 227.

CHAPTER 17:
OLIVE OIL IS NOT FOR EVERYONE: SOME BITTER VIEWS

1. "Olive Oil Quotes," ThinkExist.com, www.thinkexist.com (accessed July 13, 2007).

CHAPTER 18:
THE JOY OF COOKING WITH OLIVE OIL

1. Roe Valenti and Cal Orey, *Just Cook It! How to Get Culinary Fit . . . 1-2-3* (Lincoln, NE: iUniverse, 2004), p. 50.
2. Ibid.